get Skinny!

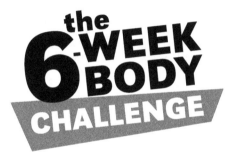

SCOTT
SCHMALTZ

New York

get skinny!

THE 6-WEEK BODY CHALLENGE

by SCOTT SCHMALTZ

ISBN 978-1-61448-123-2 Paperback
ISBN 978-1-61448-124-9 eBook
Library of Congress Control Number: 2011936588

Published by:
Morgan James Publishing
The Entrepreneurial Publisher
5 Penn Plaza, 23rd Floor
New York City, New York 10001
(212) 655-5470 Office
(516) 908-4496 Fax
www.MorganJamesPublishing.com

Cover Design by:
Rachel Lopez
rachel@r2cdesign.com

Interior Design by:
Bonnie Bushman
bbushman@bresnan.net

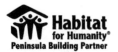

In an effort to support local communities, raise awareness and funds, Morgan James Publishing donates one percent of all book sales for the life of each book to Habitat for Humanity.
Get involved today, visit
www.HelpHabitatForHumanity.org.

dedication

If you have ever struggled with your weight, I dedicate this book to you!

foreword

My name is Heather Hansen, and I am the mother of 2 darling little girls and am married to my soul mate. I am also the owner of a successful insurance agency and a distributor for Zija International. Five years ago I started my weight loss journey and was a finalist on season three of the television show "The Biggest Loser." At that time, I weighed over 220 pounds, and my jeans were a size 22. I knew that I wasn't living my life exactly the way I wanted to, but I also didn't think that it was causing me any harm. That was until I was completely humiliated while rescuing my daughter at a McDonald's Playland.

One afternoon, when my little girl (Bella) was playing in the slides at McDonalds, she managed to get herself stuck. While rescuing Bella was my only concern, I remember feeling absolutely embarrassed. Here I was, this overweight chub, trying to wedge my way through a tiny Playland slide, hoping to rescue my little girl. The entire time, Bella kept crying out for my help, and I just kept thinking to myself, "Oh, my gosh! Please just let this be a dream. I really don't want to get stuck inside of here too."

Of course, it got worse. When I had finally gotten Bella free, I was horrified to turn around and see that some of other adults were clapping at me and snickering with one another. I felt completely humiliated. I knew that I had to make a change, but I wasn't exactly sure what I needed to do until a few weeks later when it hit me. I came up with the perfect plan while my husband and I were watching our favorite television show, "The Biggest Loser."

During the show, we noticed that all of the contestants, who had started out the season dramatically overweight, were beginning to look amazing. I was beaming with joy during that entire episode because I had just come up with my fail-proof way to lose weight: I would become a contestant on the show. Now all I had to do was get on.

The next day, I called NBC Studios to get some logistics about becoming a contestant, and I was shocked with what they told me. Tens of thousands of people would be trying out for the next season, and with all of these people trying out, I didn't stand much of a chance of getting on the show. But I wasn't going to let that stop me now. I had my fail-proof plan, and I knew what I had to do. I would simply make the most amazing audition tape possible to show them how desperately I needed their help. So, I jogged in place for hours. I raised my knees as high as I could. I did whatever I could do to show the producers, "You can count on me for the win!" Shortly after I had sent my audition tape in, they contacted me. I could hardly believe it. I was going to be a contestant!

I was extremely fortunate to get on the television show. My time at the ranch was amazing, but I also wouldn't recommend this style of weight loss for others. We worked out for a minimum of six to eight hours each and every day to lose the drastic amount of weight shown on TV, but exercising this often on your own is unrealistic.

Get Skinny! The Six-Week Body Challenge is a book that lays out a simple game plan that is so realistic that anyone can be successful. One of the things that resonates the most with me is when Scott says, "No matter where you've been or what you have done, you deserve to be successful." I understand this concept so well because my own weight loss journey has been a battle with a lot of ups and a lot of downs. If something is difficult to understand or requires too much time, you won't want to stick it out, but this book isn't difficult at all. Scott teaches the importance of consistency, and he gives you realistic weekly game plans that will help guide you in the process of losing weight and living an active lifestyle. These are things that will help you long after you're done reading the book.

I am so grateful for Scott. He took the time to write a book with no short cuts, creating something amazing that an everyday person can use to get in shape and feel great. This book is definitely worth your investment!

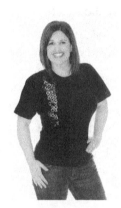

— **Heather Hansen**
Season 3 Finalist on the television show
"The Biggest Loser"
MaxTransformation.com

special message from the author

My name is Scott Schmaltz, and in addition to being the author of this book, I hope to serve as a trusted guide and friend on your journey toward health and fitness. I became a personal trainer over ten years ago because I wanted to help improve the lives other people just like you. This desire grew out of my own need to help myself during a very challenging time.

I was going through a devastating series of personal losses, and I felt like my life was falling apart. I didn't know what to do, but I knew that I needed an outlet for the anger and resentment that I was feeling.

I started exercising to help improve my mood and to help change the way that I was feeling about myself—just like so many of my other clients. It didn't take long before I started getting excited about the changes that I was making.

My health was beginning to improve, and I started helping other people around me by writing exercise programs for them, taking them through workout sessions, and being there to encourage them when they were having difficulties in their own lives. I began to feel a tremendous sense of pride in who I was and what I was becoming. This kindled a deep desire inside of me to not only want to improve my own life but to also better the lives of those around me.

I started taking all kinds of health and fitness courses, and I dedicated myself to becoming a personal trainer and a better person. Fitness became the cornerstone that made things possible. I discovered that when you take care of your health, the rest of your life naturally falls into place.

Working with clients on a personal level has become a profoundly moving experience for me. It has not only allowed me to touch the lives of hundreds of other people, but it has also given me the opportunity to help clients reach personal goals that they never thought possible.

I hope that our time together will be about more than simply getting you into shape. I also want to help you build confidence in yourself and in your ability to achieve success. I want you to know that I appreciate your commitment to change, and even though I haven't had a chance to meet you personally, I am truly grateful that you are willing to invest the time and energy necessary to make your life better by applying the principals in this book.

During the course of this **Six-Week Body Challenge**, I want you to know that it's okay to make mistakes. The most important thing that you can do to improve your health, your fitness, and your life is to learn from your mistakes and to be consistent in your efforts to change.

When I work with clients one-on-one, I make a personal commitment to helping them understand that mistakes are part of a learning process; you simply cannot have an "all or nothing" attitude. Based on my own experiences, if you become angry and pessimistic because of mistakes you've made in the past, it will begin to chip away at your self-confidence and leave you second guessing every decision that you make.

Instead, you must learn to see past your own faults and focus on what you're doing right. This will help build your sense of self-worth and give you the confidence you need to succeed.

This doesn't mean that you won't be challenged over the next six weeks. I will push you to reach for your potential, just like I expect each one of my clients to work their hardest during our workout sessions. I want to inspire you to achieve your personal best by proving to you that any negative beliefs that you hold about yourself, your health, and your body can be redefined through hard work and determination.

Even if you don't believe that you can make a radical change, believe that you can take the first step with me. The key to success is purposefully choosing to follow through on the little things that can improve your health each and every day. These small acts of consistency will turn into the positive lifestyle changes that we are all looking to achieve. *You* must be the one who is willing to take charge of your life and make a difference.

No matter what has happened in the past, and no matter where you are at right now, start over with me. You deserve to be successful!

— **Scott Schmaltz CPT, NC, HHP**

acknowledgments

I wish to express my deepest appreciations and gratitude to God for helping me to complete this book in a way that will touch the lives of those who read it. Thank you for always allowing me to know just what to say.

I wish to express the immense love and appreciation that I have for my beautiful wife Diana whose continual patience and dedication made my dream of becoming published as an author a reality. Thank you for your unwavering love and support.

I wish to express my sincerest appreciation to Rick Frishman for helping me to become published, to Scott Frishman for believing in the talents of an enthusiastic young author, to Margo Toulouse for her help and dedication to my book throughout the entire publishing process, and to the owner, David Hancock, and to the rest of staff of the Morgan James Publishing Company for their professionalism and help.

I would like to thank Heather Hansen and Greg Ladas whose support of my book from the very beginning has been an incredible blessing.

I would like to thank Greg Geiser for his legal expertise and guidance, and to Addie Zierman for her amazing and flawless work with editing my manuscript. I couldn't have done it without you.

Lastly, I would also like to express my appreciation to my family for their love and support throughout the years, and to my clients whose earnest desire to change and create a better life has helped make this book a success!

table of contents

introduction

In my years as a personal trainer, I've found that many people believe that health and fitness are synonymous. The truth is that while the two are related to one another, they're not the same thing. Being healthy is defined as being free from disease, and therefore, having a better quality of life. Conversely, being fit is defined by how well you are able to perform the different components of fitness that make up physical activity. It is these components that help you ward of sickness and disease, perform your activities of daily living (ADLs) and complete other physically demanding tasks.

For example, imagine a person who has the muscular strength needed to efficiently perform their ADLs, is somewhat flexible, and can get up a flight of stairs without becoming winded. This person would be considered physically fit. However, if that person had a diet high in saturated fat, an elevated cholesterol level and worked in a stressful environment, they would not be considered healthy.

If that same person ate a reduced fat diet, had a normal cholesterol level and properly managed their stress, he or she would be considered healthy. However, he or she would not be considered fit if they were unable to perform the physical activities listed above.

Throughout the **Six-Week Body Challenge**, my goal is to help you become more physically fit, which, in turn, will help you to become healthier and to have a better quality of life. I'll be with you every step of the way as we work to understand the different fitness components and exercise principles that make up the **Six-Week Body Challenge** and to integrate those components into your daily life.

The Five Fitness Components of the Six-Week Body Challenge

Becoming physically fit requires developing
yourself in these five different areas of fitness.

---

1. **Cardiorespiratory Fitness (CRF)** – Cardiorespiratory fitness is synonymous with several terms, including aerobic fitness and endurance as well as cardiovascular endurance. Regardless of the terminology, cardiorespiratory fitness represents your body's ability to consume and utilize oxygen for your heart, lungs and muscle tissue.

Why is Cardiorespiratory Fitness Important?

Cardiorespiratory fitness has a direct impact on your health and should be included in every fitness program. Increasing your levels of cardiorespiratory fitness will cause less stress to your heart and lungs, and this will enable you to resist disease and live a healthier life. At the same time, poor levels of CRF are linked to several health-related illnesses like obesity, heart disease, diabetes and stroke.

2. **Muscular Strength and Endurance** – Muscular strength/endurance is the amount of force your muscles can exert and sustain against resistance. Resistance includes any external object you are required to lift, such as free weights and dumbbells, household objects and your own body weight.

Why is Muscular Strength Important?

While muscular strength requirements may be subjective, muscular strength is essential for postural stability and support, joint health and performance of your daily routines. Similarly, a lack of muscular strength will lead to a decline in movement and a loss of personal independence.

3. **Flexibility** – Flexibility is measured by how freely your joints are able to move through a complete range of motion, or the distance between their bent and straight positions. Many times, maintaining flexibility is undervalued because the results are not seen in the mirror like a set of bulging biceps.

Why is Flexibility Important?

As much as good flexibility can positively impact joint health, poor flexibility can do the opposite, causing joint pain and instability, tension headaches and degeneration of the spinal joints. Poor flexibility also affects your cardiovascular endurance and muscular strength.

4. **Nutrition and Body Composition** – Body composition is your body's percentage or ratio of fat mass (fat weight) to lean mass (weight of your muscles, bones, organs and water). Body composition is directly affected by diet and exercise.

Why is Body Composition Important?

Having a poor body composition or a large percentage of fat mass to lean mass, creates an elevated risk of developing health-related illnesses like diabetes, high blood pressure and heart disease. Diet and exercise will help to reduce your body fat composition, reducing your chance of disease.

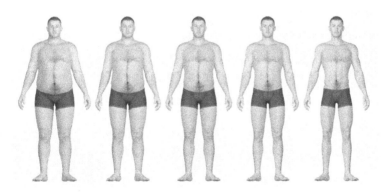

Different types of body composition ranging from 32% Body Fat (Obese) to 10% body fat (Athletic).

5. **Balance and Proprioception** – Proprioception is your unconscious ability to know where your body and its parts are spatially located, especially in relation to the ground and other fixed objects. Balance is

your ability to resist unstable forces, such as slipping on the ground. Both proprioception and balance work to keep you upright.

Why are Balance and Proprioception Important?

Proprioception is the primary means by which you learn to move your body. Without it you would have no awareness of your body and would be unable even to stand. Any exercise that requires coordination will aid in balance training and improve your proprioceptive system.

The Exercise Principles of the Six-Week Body Challenge

These basic exercise principles will help you
achieve success over the next six weeks.

Consistency

While it can seem overwhelming in the beginning, exercising on a regular basis is critical to your success in this program. Not only does consistency develop good habits, but it can also help motivate you, especially as you start to experience results. Being consistent in your efforts is the single most important thing you can do to achieve success.

To achieve the best results from the exercise programs listed in each chapter, I recommend completing the programs as they are laid out to the best of your ability. Each program should be performed a minimum of 2-3 times per week. The more consistent you are, the better your results will be.

You can perform the exercise more often if you want, but don't do them more than 4-5 times a week. When you exercise too frequently, your body doesn't have adequate time to recover, and your potential for injury increases. Similarly, as the regularity of your exercise decreases (a fewer number of exercise sessions per week), the intensity of each workout must increase to either maintain or improve your results.

• • • • • • • • • • •

Being consistent with your efforts is the single most important thing you can do to achieve success!

• • • • • • • • • • •

Depending on your fitness level and the intensity level of the workout, this may cause injury as well.

Intensity

The intensity at which you exercise reflects the amount of oxygen needed and the number of calories you will burn while working out. Exercise intensity is experienced by how hard the activity feels to you. If the intensity is too light, it will be difficult for you to achieve your desired fitness goals, and if the intensity is too hard, you increase your risk of muscle soreness, injury and burnout.

To help you achieve the best results as quickly as possible, I've created these exercise programs in a circuit training format with a moderate intensity. (The specific intensities are laid out at the beginning each of program and are expressed in a specific heart range.) The circuit training format will help improve your cardiovascular system, which is extremely important to the five components of fitness. Circuit training routines are also extremely effective at creating weight loss since total caloric expenditure is significantly higher than during other exercise routines.

Circuit training typically involves more moderate (tolerable) resistance and is a preferred method of weight loss because the exercise duration is relatively short compared to other types of fitness routines. This makes it noticeably easier to exercise at a much higher intensity than you may otherwise feel comfortable with while simultaneously allowing for improvements in your cardiovascular system.

Duration

The total amount of time you exercise in a single session is called duration. In general, the longer the duration, the more calories you burn. However, if the weight and intensity of an exercise are more than you can handle, you'll become fatigued very quickly. When this happens, you'll find that you need to rest more often during your workout and it will become difficult to burn the necessary amount of calories needed to reach your goals.

People often spend a lot of time exercising at the gym because the demands of the exercises they are performing require them to take longer rest periods. While they may have spent three hours at the gym, their body only adapted to the actual amount of contact time they had with the resistance, reducing their calorie burning potential.

The duration for circuit training tends to be very manageable. It allows you to exercise for a shorter period of time without sacrificing your ability to burn a lot of calories. You can achieve a shorter duration because your body continues moving while your contact time with the resistance gradually increases. This is done by keeping your exercises to a more moderate intensity and by reducing your total resistance.

Progressive Overload

The human body will adapt to the physical demands and stresses placed upon it. To keep you progressing within your workouts, I am going to challenge your abilities every week but not to an excess. This continual form of progression will keep things fresh and exciting as you move through the program.

I designed your programs to incrementally increase the amount of stress placed upon your body. (Each week, there will be a new program.) At the same time, I want you to feel confident in your ability to perform these exercises. Therefore, the programs will give you a base foundation to build upon for the following week.

Some of the exercises have the same basic idea but grow more complex. The intensity or order may have changed, the weight or repetitions may have increased, or some of the exercises may have been replaced with new ones. The important thing to remember is that each week builds on the previous week, giving you a skill set and a foundation to work from. I recommend that you start from the beginning on week one, day one and progress through the weeks in order.

How to Get Started

What to know and what to get before you start this program.

A key feature of the **Six-Week Body Challenge** is its flexibility. All of the programs can be done at the gym or in the comfort of your own home. Before we get started, there are a few things for you to know about how the format of each week is laid out. There are also a few items that you will need in order to complete the program.

What to Know

The format of every week will start with a transformational story about a common exercise problem and how it was overcome. We will then talk about some nutrition basics, and I will give a specific meal plan for you to follow to help you on your fitness journey.

You will also receive:

1. Cardio plan
2. Circuit training program
3. Stretching guide

Each week is laid out step-by-step so you will know exactly how to use the **Six-Week Body Challenge** to help you reach your goals.

What You'll Need

Before you get started with the **Six-Week Body Challenge**, make sure that you have access to the following things.

- A heart rate monitor. This will help you effectively achieve the right training zone or intensity for each program and get the most effective workout in the least amount of time. Make sure that your monitor includes a chest strap. This will allow you to get a continuous heart rate reading without having to stop your workout.

- A set of dumbbells ranging from 5 to 20 pounds. (Men may need a slightly larger set of dumbbells for the later weeks.)

- A medicine ball weighing 6, 8, or 10 pounds, depending on your fitness level, and a set of body bars ranging from 9 to 30 pounds.

- Cardiovascular equipment that you are comfortable using, such as an upright bike, a treadmill, and an elliptical cross-trainer machine. (If you are working out at home, you can also include activities like walking, jogging in place or running outside.)

Note: If you don't have some or all of the equipment listed above, you can purchase what you need at: *CustomWorkoutVideos.com/amazonstore.php*

It has been a great experience for me to work with so many different people over the years, and I am really looking forward to being a part of your fitness journey as well. As we start the **Six-Week Body Challenge**, please remember that if any one week is too challenging, you can always repeat that week before you move on to the next.

Now let's get started!!!

Chapter 1

true inner strength

How She Redefined Beautiful

My name is Diana, and I am a strong, powerful woman with beautiful legs. As a teenager, I remember being quite the tomboy. I loved a pick-up game of basketball, volleyball, or tennis—really anything active. I especially loved soccer, and I started getting that soccer-player-look that is commonly defined by thick, muscular legs.

On most nights after school, I would have a fast-food dinner with my family. Despite being active in sports during my free time, the junk food and the drive-thru meals started to pack on some unwanted pounds. Even though I was on the heavier side of average for a teenager, I always felt that I was a lot bigger than the rest of my friends.

When I was around 16 years old, I started to think that my legs were getting too big. I started to work out at home to my mom's Tony Little tapes in addition to playing soccer and tennis at school. I did whatever I could to help slim my legs down. I started playing any extra sports I could during my free time, even when I was away at church camp in the summers. But no matter what, my thighs kept getting bigger and more cellulite kept appearing. It got so bad that during my senior year in high school, I started to run three miles every day after school. I just kept thinking that it would help me slim down, but no matter what I did, I held at a steady 140 pounds.

I really felt depressed with how my body was turning out. I was frustrated because I thought I was doomed to be pear-shaped with big, jiggly thighs that would clap together when I would run or jog.

In college, my weight kept going up, which felt depressing because I was still working out a lot. I wanted to be healthy, but looking back, I was still eating out for most of my meals or eating pre-made microwavable food when I was in the dorms. I thought that because I was working out, it didn't matter what I'd eat. I felt justified in eating poorly.

College food was surprising delicious, and the best part was that it was served all-you-can-eat-style. I would even finish off every meal (lunch and dinner) at the cafeteria with a cookie. While I thought I was doing okay, it got to the point where my lower body became significantly out of proportion to the rest of my body.

By the end of college, my weight had ballooned out of control. I weighed well over 160 pounds, and I was only 5'2"! I was no longer able to get into my jeans, which were already a size 14. I was horrified at the idea of wearing shorts because of how disproportioned my legs were to the rest of my body, but what frightened me even more was the idea that I was going to have to start shopping at plus-sized clothing stores.

I knew I had to change my lifestyle. I thought that I was in decent shape since I been consistently exercising and running throughout college, but I joined a local gym to make the change I knew I deserved. I hired a trainer to help me get my weight back on track, and I started working out using programs that were designed for me by the author of this book.

Finally, my body started to change, but it wasn't easy at first. I had to change my way of thinking about food. My trainer gave me some nutrition guidelines to follow and helped me to watch my caloric intake.

My friends and family started noticing that I was losing weight and that I was getting more definition. But I was still frustrated with my legs and butt. I started comparing myself to, well, everybody. I'd look at other girls in front of me at the checkout line, in the magazines that I read, in the movies that I watched, or wherever I saw women that had nicer legs than me, and it made me miserable.

I felt so upset that I was working so hard and that my legs still weren't skinny or smooth like I had wanted them to be. To make it even worse, my family and even my boyfriend started to put me down. They didn't understand why I wanted to change so much. They ate whatever they wanted, and they were not all too concerned with how they looked or about their health, so they couldn't understand why I wanted to be different.

They weren't trying to be mean to me. I really believe that they just wanted me to be happy, but they were always pushing me to blow my diet and eat whatever, and they poked fun at me for monitoring what I ate. It took them a really long time to understand that this wasn't just some phase that I was going through, but it was a change that I needed to make for me, especially as obesity runs in my family.

I had a tough time when I was going through this. I would get down on myself, and I felt alone at times. I really felt like I was the only one I knew in my life who wanted something different. I remember talking to my trainer a lot during this time, and he was always patient with me and reminded me that I was doing the right thing.

He taught me about muscle-to-limb ratio and about different muscle fiber types, and I started to realize that with my petite frame and muscular legs, my legs would probably continue to change and become more sleek and defined. However, it wasn't reasonable for me to expect to look like I had always imagined I would. I had an idealized standard of beauty that I was carrying around with me, and it wasn't reality.

My trainer told me that because my frame was shorter and because I had a shorter limb-to-tendon ratio, I would have bigger-looking legs than someone who was 5'7" (the standard height of most supermodels), but that it wasn't bad. I was who I was.

He also let me in on how these models and actresses look so good. He mentioned that a lot of it had to do with genetics (i.e. the models I was looking at were all taller than me with longer limbs and posed in a way that elongated their bodies, so of course they looked skinny) and that the magazines did touch-up work to remove their bumps and blemishes before the pictures went to print. He told me that their abs and shoulders were also touched up afterward, and most importantly, that they worked extremely hard to maintain the shape they were in.

These models and actresses watched what they ate very closely, and they worked out a lot. My trainer explained that consistency was the key to everything! He told me that he believed in my potential and if I worked hard, I would achieve my goals. I just had to be patient. After all, he said that it took me well over twenty years to get out of shape, and I had to be comfortable with the fact that it would take me longer than a few weeks of being consistent before I would reach my goals. I learned that the comparison game would never make me feel better and that when you compare yourself to others, you will always feel miserable because you are comparing your worst feature to their best…so, of course you're going to lose.

I took his advice and kept working hard. I started to appreciate my legs more and more, and I learned that I had to be patient. After all, it took me a long time to get out of shape, and I had to give things time to change. I learned this from Scott. He mentioned that this was a big reason he had seen clients fail. They expected an overnight change and didn't give themselves a realistic amount of time to see the change they wanted. They set huge, unrealistic goals about what they should expect, like losing 60 pounds in a month, and then, when it didn't happen, they felt defeated and gave up.

It's been five years since I first started using Scott's workouts and about two years since I finally committed to eating right. My baby steps to becoming healthier and being more physically active have now become a permanent part of my lifestyle, and throughout this entire process, I have learned to be happy about who I am and happy about where I am at in life.

I appreciate my uniquely and perfectly designed body, and I continue to work with what I have been given in order to be the best possible me while creating my own perfect body!

I am so thankful and appreciative for my body, the legs that I have, and how my body performs. Now, I find that even when I'm watching other people, I feel confident in who I am. I appreciate the beauty that surrounds me in all its different shapes and sizes.

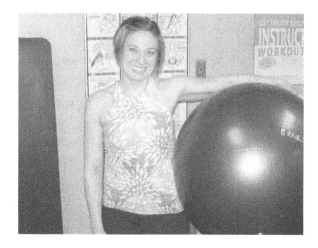

After all, each one of us is a beautiful work in progress!

Food Labels and Time Tables

Understanding Nutrition Labels and the Basics of Food Timing

Food Labels

Nutrition labels are great for helping you to lose weight because they provide you with valuable information, such as serving sizes and calories per serving.

The Break Down

Nutrition labels help you lose weight by breaking down information in the following ways:

- The **Recommended Serving Size** and the **Servings per Container** are the first items you will notice at the top of a nutrition label. A recommended serving size might be something like half of a cup. However, actual serving sizes can vary greatly and may include many different types of measurements like grams, ounces and spoons. The top of the nutrition

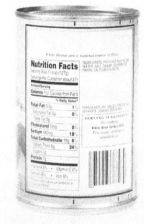

label will also list the total number of serving sizes per container.

- **Total Calories per Serving** will show you how many calories are in each serving. This is probably the most valuable piece of information listed on a nutrition label. By multiplying the number calories per serving by the total number of serving sizes, it will give you the total number of calories per container. For example: Three half cup servings multiplied by 110 calories per serving would give you 330 total calories for that food item. Always remember that the calories listed are based on one serving, and it is important that you look at the total number of servings per container before you eat the whole food item. Otherwise, you may end up consuming more calories than you need.

- The **Daily Percentage Value** will tell you how large of a percentage each nutrient is in your total daily allowance, which is almost always based on a 2,000 calorie per day diet. The nutrients that are commonly listed on a nutrition label are fat, carbohydrates, and protein, as well as major vitamins and minerals.

- The **Fat** column will show you how many total grams of fat you are consuming with each serving. Using this column will help you limit your fat intake throughout the day. As a part of your weekly meal plans, I have limited your fat intake to 25% of your total daily calories. I will be discussing fat more thoroughly in Chapter Four to help you understand my recommendations. (For every gram of fat that you eat, you will consume close to nine calories.)

- **Saturated Fats** and **Trans-Fatty Acids** are the next items on the list. For more information about these items, please reference Chapter Four.

- The **Cholesterol** column will tell you how many milligrams (mg) of cholesterol you are consuming per serving. This information is important if you are trying to lower your cholesterol.

- The **Sodium** column will tell you how many milligrams of sodium are in each serving. This will be discussed in depth in Chapter Five, but I recommend that you limit your sodium intake to 2,300 mg per day unless you have kidney disease or high blood pressure. In this case, you should limit your intake to 1,500 mg to prevent fluid retention and swelling.

- The **Carbohydrate** column will tell you how many grams of carbohydrates you are consuming with each serving size. This total is not only made up of how many grams of carbohydrates are in each serving, but also of how many grams of dietary fibers, sugars, and starches are in each serving. In the weekly meal plans that I created for this book, 50% of your total daily calories come from carbohydrates. This will give you the energy you need for your workouts without storing any extra as fat. I will discuss carbohydrates more thoroughly in Chapter Three to help you understand my recommendations. (For every gram of carbohydrate that you eat, you consume roughly four calories.)

- The **Dietary fiber** column will tell you how much fiber is in each serving. Dietary fiber is an indigestible carbohydrate and it aids in the elimination of waste. I recommend that you consume between 25-30 grams of fiber per day to help your intestines eliminate waste.

- The **Protein** column will tell you how many grams of protein are in each serving. In your weekly menus, 25% of your total daily calories come from protein. I will be discussing protein and amino acids more thoroughly in the next chapter. (For every gram of protein that you eat, you consume about four calories.)

Nutrition Timing

The timing of your food is an important aspect of your **Six-Week Body Challenge**, and it is important for maintaining the new muscle tissue that you are developing. However, I don't want you to worry about breaking your meals up into extremely small portions throughout the day to lose weight. I've created menus that are already set up to give you the right amount of meals and snacks during your day to help you lose weight. It's important to make sure that you are consistently eating throughout the day and not starving yourself.

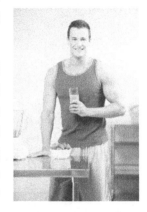

If you go too long without eating, your body will begin breaking down your muscle tissue for energy and this may cause you to feel anxious or have difficulties concentrating. You may also begin to feel dizzy and light-headed, and you may even pass out. By eating consistently throughout the day, you will be able to maintain your muscle tissue, which is positive for many reasons. Aesthetically, your muscles add to your shapely appearance while also increasing your body's metabolism.

Eat a good breakfast

Eating a good breakfast is essential in losing weight. Your first meal of the day should be highly nutritious providing you with quality carbohydrates and proteins. This will help slow the breakdown of your food and provide you with more energy throughout the day. When you get up in the morning, your body is low on carbohydrates and energy from sleeping, and when you skip breakfast, this will only get worse as your body will begin breaking down your muscle tissue to use for energy. Over time, this repeated break down of your muscle tissue will slow down your metabolic rate, making fat loss more difficult in the future.

Also, if you attempt to lose weight by skipping your first meal of the day, you will become fatigued as your brain and body run low on fuel. This is typically why people experience a "crash" around mid-morning. Trying to offset your energy levels using caffeine-based energy products only helps in the short-term. By lunchtime, your blood sugar levels will be extremely low, causing your feel shaky and irritable. It can also cause you to make poor food choices as you try and satiate your hunger. Your body will also have suppressed its ability to feel full, leading you to consume more calories than you need.

Eat a light meal two hours before bed

Before going to sleep, remember that your body will not receive nutrients for around eight hours (ten hours when you add in the extra two hours before bed.) Now is a good time to provide your body with the nutrients it needs to help prevent the breakdown of your muscle tissue. Remember that while your metabolism may slow down a bit when you go to sleep, it does not shut off altogether. Your body still needs to maintain its functions, which require energy. If you are going to bed on an empty stomach, you may have difficulties sleeping.

This is one of the causes the dreaded "midnight munchies" or snacking which is a really bad habit to start. If hunger is keeping you awake at night, the affects to your body are similar to that which occurs when you skip breakfast. Your body's ability to feel full will be suppressed, and you will make poor food choices as you try and satiate your hunger. Having a light meal two hours before bed will prevent the feeling of food sitting in your stomach while you sleep while also keeping you from experiencing hunger during the night.

Eat within a half hour to two hours before working out

To get the most out of your workout, eat a snack or a light meal 30 minutes to two hours before you exercise. This timeframe will give your food time to digest and prevent you from getting an upset stomach during your workout. It will also give you the energy you need to exercise at a more intense pace.

If you don't have a moderate amount of carbohydrates in your system (especially when exercising) your body will hit nervous system fatigue. This makes the communication signals that travel from your nervous system to your body slow down and decline in strength and makes it difficult to finish your exercise routine. This can also increase your chance of injury and may cause you to pass out during or after your workout.

Some foods you can try eating before you go to the gym are fruit, whole grain cereal with reduced-fat milk, half a sandwich, and/or a meal replacement bar. These are good choices for a pre-workout meal because they don't take long to digest, giving you a readily available supply of energy for your workout routine. Stay away from high-fat foods like a hand full of almonds or cashews since they take longer to break down before your workout and won't give you the carbohydrates you need for energy.

If you can, it's ideal to consume a larger meal 60- to 90-minutes before your workout. You will have more energy than if you just eat a snack, which will allow you to push yourself harder during your workout. It's also a good idea to eat a carbohydrate-based snack, such as a banana or a glass of orange juice, after your workout. This will help optimize your muscle recovery by refilling the sugar stores within your body. Having a carbohydrate-based snack after your workout will also help to reduce muscular soreness.

Your Weekly Menus

Each week you'll be receiving a new meal plan. I created these to help take the guess-work out of what you should be eating to lose weight and because I want to make sure that you see results from your hard work. I also don't want you to feel overwhelmed by trying to learn and apply the information from each chapter on your own, especially if it feels new to you.

Over the six weeks, you'll be able to see how the different nutrition sections and menus work together to create something that is even more powerful than weight loss alone: knowledge and understanding. Let the different nutrition sections and menus act as a guide, and by the time you are done with your **Six-Week Body Challenge**, you will have a solid foundation with which to create your own menus. You deserve to make the dream of a stronger, healthier body a reality!

Your First Menu

This Week's Menu Benefits (A Well-Balanced Diet)

There are many reasons to eat a well-balanced diet from managing your weight to controlling illnesses like diabetes. But with the term "well-balanced diet" thrown around so much, we often lose sight of the true purpose and meaning behind this lifestyle choice.

The true purpose of eating a well-balanced diet is to maintain a healthy weight and prevent disease. To consume a well-balanced diet, you must eat a wide variety of foods, leaving nothing out. Every nutrient is essential to your body and has an important role to play.

Consuming a well-balanced diet also means reducing your caloric intake and consuming only what your body needs to maintain a healthy weight. Otherwise, the creeping obesity caused by the unchecked calories will be extremely harmful to your body over time. Finally, consuming a well-balanced diet means that you have sought out the advice of your doctor to make sure that your diet will not negatively interact with any of the medications that he or she may have prescribed you.

This week's menu is teeming with delicious bell peppers and onions, farm fresh meats, and a special blend of seasonings to create a meatloaf that will satisfy even the heartiest of your appetites. This week's menu also includes plenty of rich whole grains and fresh fruits to provide your body with a wide variety of the nutrients you need to feel healthy and look great. After all, your body is worth it!

Notes on This Week's Menu

If you get tired of eating the same thing every day, you can change the order of your meals. Just make sure to stay with the same serving and portion sizes.

To keep track of your progress, it's a great idea to record your weight and your measurements at the beginning of each week. Now would also be a great time to take some starting pictures. I'm really excited to hear about your progress!

If you can't afford to buy organic or if you don't have access to an organic grocer, it's okay to make substitutions. I listed the nutritional value of the food that I picked for your menu, and when you are making substitutions (such as replacing the Thomas brand English muffin with another brand), just make sure that you are getting as close to the same nutritional value per serving as possible.

Also, if you are having difficulties finding some of the food items on your menu, they can be purchased through my catalog store: *CustomWorkoutVideos. com/amazonstore.php.* Availabilities may vary depending on Amazon.

<u>Special Entrée of the Week</u>

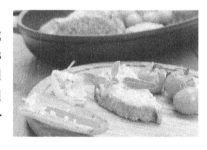

Bison Mexican Meatloaf is an exciting entree teeming with delicious bell peppers and onions, farm fresh meats, and a special blend of seasonings that combines traditional meatloaf with a South of the border flavor that is sure to please!

This recipe is available for only $0.99 at:
CustomWorkoutVideos.com/catalog/index.php

Women's Menu: Week One

Breakfast	Serving Size	Calories	Grams Protein Carbs, Fat	Comments
English Muffin	0.5 muffin (1oz)	60 cal	2g protein, 12.5g carbs, 0.5g fat	based on Thomas Muffins
Creamy Peanut Butter	0.5 tbsp (0.6oz)	47 cal	2g protein, 1.75g carbs, 4g fat	based on natural creamy Jif peanut butter
Chocolate Almond Milk	0.75 cups (6oz)	70 cal	1g protein, 12g carbs, 2g fat	based on Blue Diamond brand milk
Whey Protein (lactose free)	1 scoop (0.6oz)	55 cal	10g protein, 4g carbs, 0g fat	based on Bio-Chem Berry Whey Protein

Snacks	Serving Size	Calories	Grams Protein Carbs, Fat	Comments
Raspberry Greek Yogurt	1 cup (6oz)	140 cal	14g protein, 20g carbs, 0g fat	based on no-fat Chobani brand yogurt

Lunch	Serving Size	Calories	Grams Protein Carbs, Fat	Comments
Rosemary Olive Oil Bread	2 slices (2.8oz)	200 cal	8g protein, 40g carbs, 2g fat	based on Rudi's Organic (can be traded for wheat, any)
Deli Meat Roast Beef or Smoked Turkey	1 serving (2oz)	60 cal	12g protein, 0g carbs, 3g fat	based on using Applegate Farms deli meat

Swiss or Sharp Cheddar Cheese Slice	1 slice (1oz)	110 cal	7g protein, 0g carbs, 9g fat	based on Trader Joes sharp cheddar cheese
Butterhead Lettuce	2 slices (0.4oz)	<1cal	0g protein, <1g carbs, 0g fat	based on an average organic brand
Roma Tomato	4 slices (2.8oz)	14 cal	<1g protein, 3g carbs, 0g fat	based on an average organic brand
Yellow Mustard	1-2 tsp (0.2oz)	0 cal	0g protein, <1g carbs, 0g fat	based on French's classic yellow mustard

Snacks	**Serving Size**	**Calories**	**Grams Protein Carbs, Fat**	**Comments**
Granola Bar	0.5 package (1 bar)	80 cal	3g protein, 13g carbs, 2g fat	based on Nature Valley brand (apple crisp)
Orange or Apple	1 medium (4.6oz)	60 cal	1g protein, 16g carbs, 0g fat	based on an average organic fresh brand

Dinner	**Serving Size**	**Calories**	**Grams Protein Carbs, Fat**	**Comments**
Jasmine Rice (for Spanish rice, add taco seasoning)	0.33 cup (2.4oz)	240 cal	6g protein, 51g carbs, 3g fat	based on Lundberg's (uncooked Jasmine rice)
*Bison Mexican Meatloaf	1 serving (4oz)	202 cal	25g protein, 7g carbs, 9g fat	Custom Workout Videos.com brand

Men's Menu: Week One

Breakfast	Serving Size	Calories	Grams Protein Carbs, Fat	Comments
English Muffin	1 muffin (2oz)	120 cal	4g protein, 25g carbs, 1g fat	based on Thomas Muffins
Creamy Peanut Butter	1 tbsp (0.6oz)	95 cal	4g protein, 3.5g carbs, 8g fat	based on Natural Creamy Jif
Chocolate Almond Milk	1.5 cups (12oz)	140 cal	2g protein, 24g carbs, 4g fat	based on Blue Diamond brand milk
Whey Protein (lactose free)	1 scoop (0.6oz)	55 cal	10g protein, 4g carbs, 0g fat	based on Bio-Chem Berry Whey Protein

Snacks	Serving Size	Calories	Grams Protein Carbs, Fat	Comments
Granola Bar	0.5 package (1 bar)	80 cal	3g protein, 13g carbs, 2g fat	based on Nature Valley brand (apple crisp)
Raspberry Greek Yogurt	1 cup (6oz)	140 cal	14g protein, 20g carbs, 0g fat	based on no-fat Chobani brand Greek yogurt

Lunch	Serving Size	Calories	Grams Protein Carbs, Fat	Comments
Rosemary Olive Oil Bread	2 slices (2.8oz)	200 cal	8g protein, 40g carbs, 2g fat	based on Rudi's Organic (can be traded for wheat, any)
Deli Meat Roast Beef or Smoked Turkey	1.5 servings (3oz)	90 cal	18g protein, 0g carbs, 4.5g fat	based on Applegate Farms deli meat

	1 slice (1oz)	110 cal	7g protein, 0g carbs, 9g fat	based on Trader Joes sharp cheddar cheese
Swiss or Sharp Cheddar Cheese Slice	1 slice (1oz)	110 cal	7g protein, 0g carbs, 9g fat	based on Trader Joes sharp cheddar cheese
Butterhead Lettuce	2 slices (0.4oz)	<1cal	0g protein, <1g carbs, 0g fat	based on an average organic brand
Roma Tomatoes	4 slices (2.8oz)	14 cal	<1g protein, 3g carbs, 0g fat	based on an average organic brand
Yellow Mustard	1-2 tsp (0.2oz)	0 cal	0g protein, <1g carbs, 0g fat	based on French's classic yellow mustard

Snacks	Serving Size	Calories	Grams Protein Carbs, Fat	Comments
Granola Bar	0.5 package (1 bar)	80 cal	3g protein, 13g carbs, 2g fat	based on Nature Valley brand (apple crisp)
Orange or Apple	1 large (6.5oz)	85 cal	1g protein, 22g carbs, 0g fat	based on an average organic brand

Dinner	Serving Size	Calories	Grams Protein Carbs, Fat	Comments
Jasmine Rice (for Spanish rice, add taco seasoning)	0.33 cup (2.4oz)	240 cal	6g protein, 51g carbs, 3g fat	based on Lundberg's (uncooked Jasmine rice)
*Bison Mexican Meatloaf	1.5 servings (6oz)	303 cal	37.5g protein, 10.5g carbs, 13.5g fat	Custom Workout Videos.com brand

Your First Cardio Plan

Understanding the Format and Maximizing Your Time

Before we start, let's take a moment to talk about how your weekly cardio programs will be structured.

Maximizing Your Time

Because cardiovascular training has a direct impact on your health (see Introduction) and because cardio is one of the five major components of fitness, I want to make sure you're doing some cardiovascular exercise every week. However, I'll streamline your efforts to make this easier for you so that you don't have to spend your entire week exercising!

The standard recommendations for cardiovascular exercise are to perform some type of cardio 3-5 days per week at a moderate to a moderately high intensity. Staying at the lower end of the spectrum (fewer days per week) will allow you to simply maintain your endurance levels. Moving toward the upper end of the spectrum (more days per week) will help you to achieve weight loss and cardiovascular improvement. However, following the conventional guidelines can be really boring and time consuming.

To make sure you are getting the most benefit while streamlining your efforts, I designed each of your fitness routines to include a cardiovascular component. (This is also one of the reasons why I choose the circuit training format.) Doing the exercise routines in each chapter a minimum of 2-3 times per week will give you the same benefits of performing conventional cardiovascular exercise 2-3 days per week. You'll also experience a considerable amount of fat loss while making these improvements to your cardiovascular system.

All you need to do is wear your heart rate monitor and follow the recommendations for the intensity (heart rate training zones) listed in each program. In the cardio sections, I'll also give you a broader breakdown of the intensities listed in your exercise program as well as for the small amounts of additional cardiovascular exercise I want you to do with each program. These additional breakdowns will give you a better overview of what you are trying to achieve each week.

Understanding the Format

In addition to the cardiovascular benefits you are receiving from each circuit training program, you should still do a little cardio before and after each program. Every week, I'll describe a new cardiovascular exercise. This will help keep things fun and exciting!

This may seem confusing since I've combined your cardio exercise with your fitness exercises, and since I said that as long as you're following the recommended intensities, you are fine. However, performing 7-10 minutes of cardio before your program allows for proper oxygenation of your muscle tissue. This acts as your warm up and helps to prevent injury.

You should also perform 10-15 minutes of cardio exercise when you're done with your program. This will increase your calorie burn while improving your cardiovascular system. Adding some cardio to the end of your program will also help to significantly reduce muscular soreness in the days that follow your workout and prevent injury. Lastly, it helps to prevent blood from pooling when you are done working out, which may be experienced as heaviness in your extremities.

Following these cardio recommendations each week will give you a minimum of seven minutes of cardio before and ten minutes of cardio after your program. This keeps you pretty close to the conventional recommendations of 20-30 minutes of cardio 3-5 times per week, and it doesn't even count the cardio you are getting from the circuit training itself! This puts you well within the conventional guidelines while majorly increasing your calorie burning potential per workout.

If you want, you can do an extra day of cardio every week outside of your circuit training to accelerate your results, but don't do more than one or two extra workouts a week. More than that may lead to excessive muscle soreness, exercise burnout and increased potential for an overuse injury.

Note: Even with the extra time for the cardio along with the circuit training and stretching that makes up your complete routine, you are really only exercising for just over an hour 2-3 times per week. This is incredibly streamlined, particularly considering we're hitting all of the five components of fitness. This format also keeps you from having to become a gym rat just to live a healthier lifestyle.

Your First Cardio Program

Your cardio program for the first week utilizes the upright bike. (Remember, your cardio program will change every week to give you the most diverse and interesting program possible.)

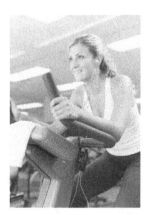

Warm Up (7-10 min) Begin by completing 7-10 minutes of cardio on the upright bike before you start your workout routine. Your heart rate should be between 100-120 bpm (beats per minute)—about 50-55% of your maximum heart rate. Working within this heart rate zone will help warm up your body and improve your circulatory system.

Cardio: End of Program (10-15 min) Complete 10-15 minutes of cardio after your program. This time is strictly allotted for cardio, so make sure to your heart rate up between 140-160 bpm. This is closer to 60-70% of your maximum heart rate. Working out in this heart rate zone will improve your heart and lungs while keeping you in a fat-burning zone. (As your cardio system gets stronger, this zone will start to change.)

When exercising at this intensity, you should still be able to speak, but in only small sentences. Your rate of breathing will become much heavier than during your warm-up. These physiological cues will help reinforce when you are training at the right intensity.

Now, let's get going!

Get Motivated! Workout One

What to Know

Your first program is designed to introduce you to circuit training. Circuit training is an extremely effective way to lose weight because you burn more calories than when you use other types of exercise routines. The circuit training routine is designed specifically to promote weight loss.

Unlike other exercise routines, circuit training allows you to burn more fat and total calories in a shorter period of time since you're working out at a higher intensity. Circuit training also utilizes lighter resistances than other types of workout routines, making it easier for you to push yourself at more vigorous pace. Finally, the overall length of time in which you are working out is relatively short. These qualities make it easier for you to push yourself harder than you may otherwise feel comfortable. As an added bonus, circuit training improves your cardiovascular system because you are using more oxygen during your workout!

When you exercise at a more vigorous pace, you burn more fat and total calories than when you perform less intense activities. An example of this can be seen by comparing similar exercises: walking and running. A 150-pound person walking for 20 minutes (3mph) will burn 100 calories, with 65 of those calories being burned as fat. However, if the same person doubles their intensity by running (6mph) for 20 minutes instead of walking, he or she will burn 250 calories in the same period of time with 100 of those calories being burned as fat.

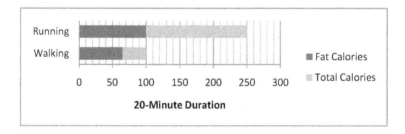

Thus, simply by increasing your intensity, you burn more calories as fat while burning more calories in total, increasing your ability to lose weight. Also, exercising at a more vigorous pace will temporarily increase your body's metabolism afterward, allowing you to burn more fat even after your workout is done.

In addition to helping you lose weight, your first workout routine is designed to help you fix your posture so you will look leaner and more sculpted. I'll explain these benefits more thoroughly in the next chapter.

The exercises in the following routine should be completed one after the other with little-to-no rest in between. Perform each of the exercises for the specified number of repetitions, then move to the next exercise. Once you have completed all the exercises, you have completed one circuit.

If at any point during your routine you experience one or more of the following symptoms, please stop exercising and allow yourself adequate time to catch your breath and reduce your heart rate before you continue:

1. Inability to focus attention or catch your breath
2. Dizziness, lightheadedness or extreme paleness in the skin
3. Stitching in the sides, stomach cramps, nausea, or chest pain

---

Get Motivated! Workout One

Let's Get Started!!!

Get Motivated! Workout One

Protocol and Order:

- **(Warm Up)** Perform 7-10 minutes of cardio on the upright bike before you start your routine, keeping your heart rate between 100-120 bpm.
- **(Exercise)** Perform *three to four* circuits in order, keeping your heart rate between 130-150 bpm.
- **(Cardio)** Perform 10-15 minutes of cardio after your program on the upright bike with your heart rate between 140-160 bpm.
- **(Stretch)** Cool down using the stretches provided in this guide.

Duration: Week One

Days per week: 2-3 (Leave 24 hours between sessions)

Exercise Reps: 10-12 or 12-15, depending on exercise

Load: Body weight or 30-40% 1 rep max

Circuits: 3-4

Rest interval: 15-30 seconds between exercises; 3-4 minutes between circuits

Equipment: Women: Two 5-8 lb dumbbells and two 8-12 lb dumbbells

Men: Two 8-10 lb dumbbells, two 10-12 lb dumbbells, and two 12-15 lb dumbbells

Note: The last few reps on each exercise should be taxing. When you can comfortably perform the number of repetitions suggested, increase your weight.

Romanian Deadlift # 1

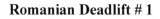

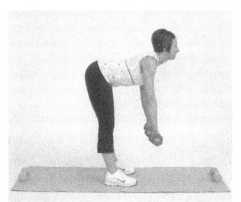 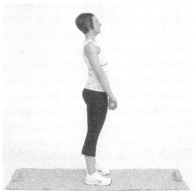

a. Start with your feet shoulder-width apart. Bend over at the waist until your torso is parallel with the floor, and look up to keep your head in alignment with the rest of your spine.

b. Stick your butt up and out, keeping your chest up. Extend the dumbbells downward and in line with your shoulders (palms facing your legs).

c. While maintaining a flat back, gently thrust your hips forward, contracting your hamstrings and glutes until your body is upright with your hips in line with the rest of your spine. Return to the starting position and repeat.

Special Instructions:

Maintain only a slight bend in the knees to prevent strain to your lower back. Throughout the exercise, avoid rounding your back, as this can cause injury.

Perform: 10-12 repetitions
Women: 8-10 lb dumbbells (each hand)
Men: 12-15 lb dumbbells (each hand)

Modified (Sumo Squat) Deadlift # 2

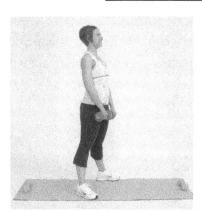 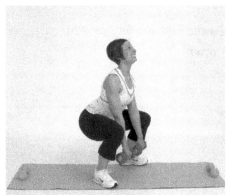

a. **(Part 1)** Stand with your feet slightly wider than your shoulder-width apart, and turn your toes out until your knees are in line with your hips. Squat down, sticking your butt out while elevating your chest to avoid rounding your back. (Rounding your back can cause injury.)

b. As you bend down, hold the dumbbells between your legs, letting your arms move along the inside of your legs. Continue to squat until the points of your elbows touch the inside of your thighs.

c. **(Part 2)** Keeping your chest elevated, exhale and gently thrust your hips forward while contracting your hamstrings and glutes until your body is upright. Keep the back in a flat position as you lift off the floor and extend through the heels. Repeat.

Perform: 10-12 repetitions
Women: 8-12 lb dumbbells (each hand)
Men: 12-15 lb dumbbells (each hand)

Bent Over Row # 3

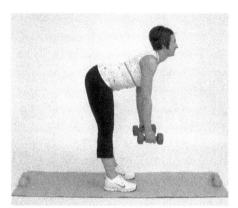 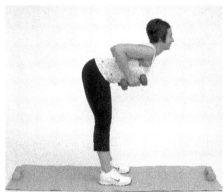

a. Bend over at the waist so your torso is parallel with the floor and your feet are shoulder-width apart.

b. Keep a slight bend in your knees, stick your butt out, keep your chest up, and extend the dumbbells downward (palms facing each other).

c. While maintaining a flat back, raise your arms by bending at your elbows (while contracting your shoulders) until your shoulders are completely abducted.

d. Hold this position for a second and return until your arms are extended and your shoulders are stretched forward. Repeat.

Perform: 10-12 repetitions
Women: 8-12 lb dumbbells (each hand)
Men: 12-15 lb dumbbells (each hand)

Bicep Curl to Press # 4

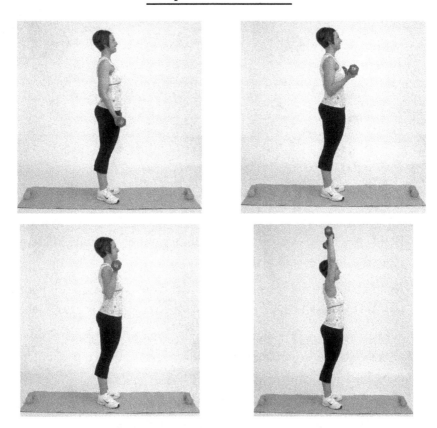

a. **(Part 1)** Hold a dumbbell in each hand with a soft grip. Weights should be at your sides with your palms facing upward.

b. Stand with your back upright and feet together in a V-shape like you are standing at attention with your legs and glutes contracted. Keep your back upright, shoulders relaxed and elbows in.

c. Slowly raise the weights by bending your elbows inward until your knuckles are 3-4 inches away from your shoulders. Then, turn your palms until they're facing outward.

d. **(Part 2)** Look up and inhale while pressing to keep your spine straight. (This will help you avoid arching your back.) Stop when your arms are extended straight overhead. Keep your wrists, shoulders and elbows in a straight line.

e. Exhale and slowly lower the weights back to your starting position in the same way that you pressed up; back down to the shoulder press, then back down to the bicep curl. Repeat.

Perform: 12-15 repetitions
Women: 5-8 lb dumbbells (each hand)
Men: 10-12 lb dumbbells (each hand)

Lateral Shoulder Raise to Stop Sign # 5

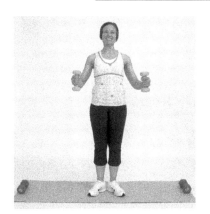 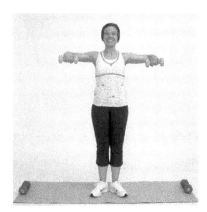

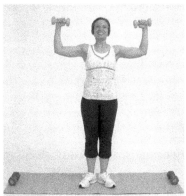

a. **(Part 1)** Stand with your back upright and your feet together in a V-shape, legs and glutes contracted. Keep your back upright, shoulders relaxed and elbows bent.

b. Start with your elbows bent and in towards your sides but not touching. They should be about 2-3 inches from your sides during the beginning and end of the exercise to fully engage the medial deltoid. This starting and ending position looks similar to a bench press.

c. Slowly raise your weights by lifting your elbows straight out to your sides until they are in line with your shoulders.

d. **(Part 2)** Look up, inhale, and slowly rotate your arms backward like a crossing guard raising a stop sign until your first resistance barrier (looking up helps to avoid arching your back).

e. Exhale and slowly rotate your arms back to your bench press position. Drop your elbows back down to your sides until they are 2-3 inches from your sides. Repeat.

Perform: 10-12 repetitions
Women: 5-8 lb dumbbells (each hand)
Men: 8-10 lb dumbbells (each hand)

Your First Stretching Routine

Now that you're done with your workout, let's cool down!

What to Know

Flexibility is measured by how freely your joints are able to move through a complete range of motion (ROM), or the distance between their bent and straight positions.

Increasing your body's flexibility will not only help to improve the overall health of your joints, but will also help to maintain your independence throughout your lifetime, especially as you age.

The type of stretching that you will be doing each week at the end of your workout routines is called static stretching. This type of stretching should always be done at the end of your workout routine because stretching a cold muscle can cause injury.

When you stretch, you should avoid bouncing or ballistic movements, as these can injure or tear the muscle that you are attempting to stretch. For the following routine, you will want to find a comfortable depth where the muscle is being stretched, and then hold for 30 seconds before relaxing.

Note: Holding a stretch should never hurt. If it does, you're either not stretching the muscle correctly, not sufficiently warmed up, or you're attempting to stretch the muscle too far. If this happens, slowly relax the muscle, wait for a bit, and then try again.

Your Stretching Routine for the First Week

Perform each stretch for 30 seconds and then slowly relax for up to ten seconds before repeating. Remember that you will need to do each stretch twice before you move onto the next, and be aware that if you release the stretch too quickly, you can cause your muscles to tighten (spasm) instead of loosen.

Hamstring Stretch

- Keep your back upright.
- Straighten one leg while tucking the other in.
- Lean forward with your back upright until you are comfortably stretching the backside of your leg.

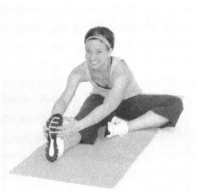

Stretching Benefits:

Tight hamstring muscles can cause back pain by pulling your pelvis out of its normal alignment.

Perform: 2 sets of 1 repetition
Sides: Both
Hold stretch for 30 seconds.

Sitting Piriformis Stretch

- Sit up straight and cross one leg over the other.
- Grab your knee with your opposite arm.
- Pull your leg towards your chest.

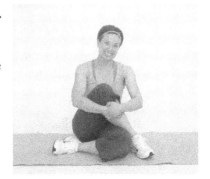

Stretching Benefits:

Tight piriformis muscles can pull your pelvis out of its normal alignment, which can put pressure on your sciatic nerves causing pain.

Perform: 2 sets of 1 repetition
Sides: Both
Hold stretch for 30 seconds.

Downward Dog (Calf) Stretch

- Start on all fours with hands and knees shoulder-width apart.

- Breathe and push the palms of your hands into the floor. Drop your shoulders as you breathe.

- Slowly straighten your legs upward, push your pelvis towards the back wall, and lift your head up. For beginners, it is okay to have a slight bend in your knees.

Stretching Benefits:

Tight calf muscles can put pressure on your knees and pelvis causing pain and irritation.

Perform: 2 sets of 1 repetition
Hold stretch for 30 seconds.

Ball-Lying Chest Stretch

- Lie with your back on the ball.

- Roll down until your head and neck are fully supported.

- Relax your hips and let your arms fall out to your sides.

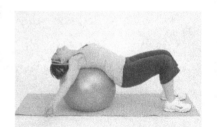

Stretching Benefits:

Tight chest muscles can cause an Upper Cross Syndrome or rounded shoulders, which can lead to bursitis, a shoulder impingement or a rotator cuff injury.

Perform: 2 sets of 1 repetition
Hold stretch for 30 seconds.

Arm-Shoulder (Towel) Stretch

- Grab a hand towel and extend one hand down your back with your hand in line with your spine, pointing down.

- Use the other hand to reach behind your back to grab the towel.

- Gently pull down on the towel, and then repeat, pulling up on the towel with the other hand.

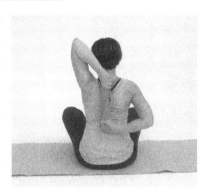

Stretching Benefits:

Tight arm and shoulder muscles can cause neck tension, headaches and can put pressure on your rotator cuff muscles and tendons.

Perform: 2 sets of 1 repetition
Sides: Both
Hold stretch for 30 seconds.

Scalene Neck Stretch

- Grab your left arm behind your back with your right hand and pull down.

- Look straight ahead and lean your head to your right side like you're trying to touch your ear to your shoulder.

- Avoid lifting your shoulder while stretching.

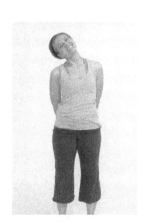

get skinny!

Stretching Benefits:

Tight scalene muscles can clamp down on your subclavian arteries, restricting the blood flow to your arms and hands and causing numbness, pain, and coldness in your arms and hands.

Perform: 2 sets of 1 repetition
Sides: Both
Hold stretch for 30 seconds.

Chapter 2

committed to change

One Woman's Journey from Thick to Thin

My name is Betty, and I have been overweight for a long time. I was fit when I was younger because my husband and I enjoyed being active, but a lot of this changed when we started to have a family. As we had children, the time that I had for myself slowly dwindled away until it was difficult to be active or have any time for myself at all.

I don't regret having a family for a second, but it did make it difficult to watch what I was eating and to be active. There were so many nights of coming home from work, then quickly getting dinner ready for two very active boys before rushing them off to their after school sports activities.

It got to a point where it was just so much easier to have meals on the fly than it was to always try to prepare a wholesome meal, even though I did do my best, especially on nights that I didn't need to rush out the door right after work.

As my boys got a little older, it started to get easier for my husband and me to go out. We did some active things, like going for walks or for motorcycle rides, but we also really enjoyed going out for drinks with our friends. I didn't realize that not eating enough of the right things throughout the week, and then eating a lot of easily prepared meals with some drinks on the weekend was going to add up to so much weight gain.

After years of this routine, I had gotten to a place where I was becoming unhappy with the person who I saw in the mirror. I wasn't unhappy with who I was as a person, but I was becoming really unhappy with how I looked and felt.

I started to look for a magic pill to help me change. I was hoping for a simple and easy solution where I didn't have to work very hard. I think that this was pretty normal for someone in my situation, and I spent so much of my time taking care of my family that I didn't have a lot of time to take care of myself. So, a weight-loss pill seemed like it was going to be an easy solution.

Over the next few years, I spent a lot of time and money trying different fad diets and bogus weight-loss products, thinking that they would be the key for me. I became really frustrated when I wasn't losing the weight that I had wanted to. I had even started to think that maybe I wasn't supposed to lose weight, and I was going to have to live with being overweight for the rest of my life. It hadn't occurred to me that the problem was with my lifestyle.

This was around the time when I met Scott. I had joined a gym close to my house. I wasn't quite ready to give up on my desire to lose weight, and the only thing that I hadn't tried was committing myself to eating right and exercising on a consistent basis. I also knew that if I was going to be successful, I was going to need some serious motivation. I would need someone who would hold me accountable to getting to the gym.

During my first session with Scott, he told me that I was going to have to make a commitment to making positive changes to my life. I was going to need a reason why I wanted to change, outside of my immediate goal of looking better in the mirror. When I hit my short-term goal, I would have to have a reason to keep working out.

This wasn't going to be a problem; I was making these changes for *me*. I wanted to improve my endurance. I was so sick of having to take the elevator at work because I didn't have the stamina to get up the stairs. I wanted to have more energy throughout the day; I was so tired of feeling exhausted all the time. Most importantly, I wanted to be able to enjoy spending time with my husband, especially as my boys were starting to get older and would be out of the house soon. I wanted to be able to do all the fun activities that we loved like going for walks and hiking. We were also planning to take a trip to sunny Texas in a few months, and I wanted to look good as we lounged around on the beach.

I won't lie: in the beginning, it was tough. Really tough. Scott constantly challenged me to improve my exercise habits, and he pushed me to develop better eating habits too. I always thought that if you wanted to lose weight, you needed to eat less, but I soon realized that I wasn't eating enough to lose weight. If this sounds confusing, don't worry...I was confused too.

When I first started training with Scott, I wasn't eating much of anything. In fact, I was kind of starving myself. I thought that if I was going to be successful losing weight, I needed to severely restrict my calorie intake. This only made things worse. When I got really hungry, I would binge on anything I could find, which usually meant foods that weren't good for me. I would also snack on candy and junk food throughout the day because I thought that snacking would help me avoid eating bigger meals, reducing my calorie intake. While a few healthy snacks throughout the day are good, lots of chocolate candies aren't.

I had to not only eat more of the right things, but I also had to keep track of what I was eating so I wouldn't overdo the bad things by underestimating my portion sizes. The key for me was really about learning to eat more of the right foods, not just eating less food altogether.

Scott also pushed me to find a weight-loss support group and a workout buddy who could help keep me accountable to my diet and exercise goals outside of time together at the gym. I have not only found a weight-loss support group, but the best part is, I have also found a group of girls at work who like to go walking during their lunch breaks. This has been so helpful because on days when I feel like being lazy, they really help to push me out the door. Now, I walk an average of 10,000 steps a day!

I really feel great about all of the changes that I have been making, especially as I have no problem making these changes a regular part of my lifestyle. I have lost well over 30 pounds and a total of 7 inches from my arms, waist, and thighs. Plus, all of my co-workers and friends are starting to call me skinny. Everyone has been noticing!

If I can do it, I know you can too! You just have to be committed to making a change.

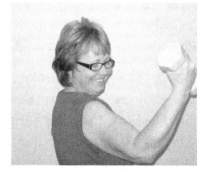

The Make-Up and Break-Up of Protein

Understanding Protein and What it Does for the Body.

Protein

It's easy to get excited about protein. Protein is vital for every cell in your body. Protein aids in the growth and repair of muscle tissue, and it is an important building block of your body's tissues like bones and cartilage. Protein is also amazing because it helps regulate your hormone levels, making you feel better. So, what is protein?

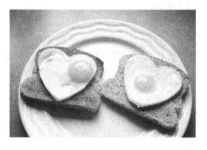

The Make-Up and Break-Up

Similar to carbohydrates and fat, protein is a "macronutrient", and unlike vitamins and minerals, also called "micronutrients," the body needs large quantities of protein on a daily basis. Protein is made up of several different structural units called amino acids, and these amino acids are either converted into fuel or built into proteins to aid the body in the processes listed above. Of the 20 different recognized types of amino acids, there are two kinds:

Essential: These amino acids cannot be made by the body, and must be supplied either through diet or through supplementation. There are a total of eight different amino acids that are essential to the body.

Nonessential: These amino acids are made by the body or from other amino acids.

Proteins are determined to be complete or incomplete based how many of the eight essential amino acids are in the food that you like to eat, either animal or plant based. Regardless of the type of protein that you like to eat, it is important that you consume all of the eight essential amino acids.

Animal proteins like chicken and fish contain all of the essential amino acids your body needs for maintenance and repair, while vegetable-based proteins do not. Plant-based proteins are generally considered to be incomplete because they are missing one or more of the essential amino acids. However, it is easy to overcome this deficiency by eating a variety of different plant-based proteins.

Vegetable proteins are also beneficial for the body because they contain large amounts of water and fiber, helping to reduce your cholesterol levels.

Over-Consumption (Organ Stress)

Many people tend to consume more than the amount of protein required for their daily needs. This can lead to many health-related issues like stress to the digestive organs and liver, loss of water weight through ketosis (leading to dehydration and kidney stones), and more acidity in the blood, which can cause calcium loss in the bones.

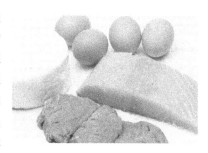

Note: The rapid weight loss in diets like the Atkin's Diet is often due to water loss from excessive proteins and to not consuming enough carbohydrates to help replenish the water supplies in the body.

How Much Protein Do You Need?

On average, you need to consume between 15 and 30% of your total daily calories from protein. The flexibility in this range allows you to determine how much protein you should eat based on your level of physical activity. In **The Six-Week Body Challenge**, I have designed your menus so that 25% of your total calories come from protein.

For Men: Each week, your daily menu contains a total of 1,800 calories, 25% of those calories coming from protein. This means that you are consuming a total of 450 calories of protein each and every day. From there, it is really easy to convert that number into grams. Since there are four calories per gram of protein, we simply divide 450 by four, which works out to roughly 113 grams of protein per day.

● ● ● ● ● ● ● ● ● ●
Protein Activity Range:
15-20%: sedentary
to low activity
20-25%: moderately active
25-30%: highly active
● ● ● ● ● ● ● ● ● ●

For Women: Each week, your daily menu contains a total of 1,400 calories, and because you are also consuming 25% of your total calories from protein, your total daily intake of protein needs to equal 350 calories. To convert this into grams, divide your intake of 350 calories by four. This means that you need to consume roughly 88 grams of protein per day to maintain, repair, and build new muscle tissue.

Note: This section and the other nutrition sections in this book are here to help you understand the *how* and *why* of your weekly menus. For now, make sure to use your pre-made meal plans each week so you can lose weight. Then, when you are finished with your body challenge, you will have not only lost weight, but you will also understand how to create your own menus based on your own individual needs!

Choose Your Proteins Wisely

Many nutrition experts (including myself) recommend getting your dietary protein from the following sources:

- **Lean Meats:** Lean meats such as skinless chicken or ground turkey offer less saturated fats and cholesterol. Some lean meats, like fish, also contain the added bonus of heart-healthy omega-3 fatty acids.
- **Beans (Legumes):** Beans contain more protein than other vegetable proteins and are loaded with fiber, which helps you feel full. To help with the gassy side-effects, soak and boil your beans before eating.
- **Whole grains:** Whole grains contain lots of fiber and protein and plenty of Vitamin B.
- **Nuts:** Nuts are great for the body and are a good source of fiber, but watch out: they do contain a lot of fat—even though it's the good kind.

Your Second Menu

This Week's Menu Benefits (Increasing Your Protein Intake)

Increasing your protein intake will help your body fight off illness and disease by keeping your immune system healthy and strong. It also helps build firm, capable muscles to give you the quality of life that you deserve!

This week's menu is full of fresh fruit and vegetables, hearty nuts, and rich-whole grains to energize your batteries. It also offers a mouthwatering sweet and sour chicken meal that is sure to please.

Notes on This Week's Menu

Tired of eating the same thing every day? It's okay to change the order of your meals. Just make sure to stay with the same serving and portion sizes. Also, remember to record your weight and measurements at the beginning of the week and to take some follow-up pictures.

Some of the food items on your menu are available through my catalog store: *CustomWorkoutVideos.com/amazonstore.php*. Availabilities may vary depending on Amazon.

Special Entrée of the Week

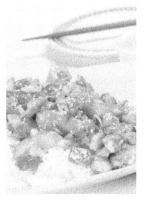

Sweet and Sour Chicken offers bold chunks of fresh red and yellow peppers, mouthwatering pieces of pineapple, and farm fresh chicken in a sweet and sour

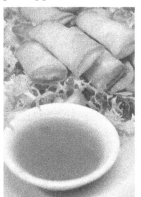

sauce. This delicious recipe gives you a high-protein, low-fat meal that is sure to please!

Sweet and Sour Sauce is 100% natural and homemade and is excellent for traditional Chinese cuisine. It also makes the perfect dipping sauce for chicken wings and fresh vegetables and is fantastic as a glazing sauce for meats like turkey and ham!

Both recipes are available for only $0.99 each at:
CustomWorkoutVideos.com/catalog/index.php

Women's Menu: Week Two

Breakfast	Serving Size	Calories	Grams Protein Carbs, Fat	Comments
Instant Oatmeal	1 pack (1.2oz)	130 cal	3g protein, 27g carbs, 2g fat	based on Quaker oatmeal (strawberry)
Blueberry Greek Yogurt	1 cup (6oz)	140 cal	14g protein, 20g carbs, 0g fat	based on no-fat Chobani brand yogurt

Snacks	Serving Size	Calories	Grams Protein Carbs, Fat	Comments
Banana	1 medium (4.2oz)	83 cal	1g protein, 21g carbs, 0.5g fat	based on an average organic brand

Lunch	Serving Size	Calories	Grams Protein Carbs, Fat	Comments
Pita Pocket Bread	0.5 pocket (1.2oz)	80 cal	3g protein, 16g carbs, 0g fat	based on Kangaroo Pita Pockets
Deli Meat Smoked Turkey or Roast Beef	1 serving (2oz)	60 cal	12g protein, 0g carbs, 3g fat	based on Applegate Farms deli meat
Sharp Cheddar or Swiss Cheese Slice	1 slice (1oz)	110 cal	7g protein, 0g carbs, 9g fat	based on Trader Joes sharp cheddar cheese
Butterhead Lettuce	2 slices (0.4oz)	1cal	0g protein, 1g carbs, 0g fat	based on an average organic brand
Roma Tomatoes	4 slices (2.8oz)	14 cal	1g protein, 3g carbs, 0g fat	based on an average organic brand
Yellow Mustard	1-2 tsp (0.2oz)	0 cal	0g protein, 1g carbs, 0g fat	based on French's classic yellow mustard

Snacks	Serving Size	Calories	Grams Protein Carbs, Fat	Comments
Rosemary Olive Oil Crackers	6 crackers (1oz)	120 cal	3g protein, 20g carbs, 4g fat	based on Triscuit's brand
Sharp Cheddar or Swiss Cheese Slice	1 slice (1oz)	110 cal	7g protein, 0g carbs, 9g fat	based on Trader Joes sharp cheddar cheese
Sweet Bell Peppers	10 strips (1oz)	5 cal	0.5g protein, 1g carbs, 0g fat	based on average organic brand (any color)

Dinner	Serving Size	Calories	Grams Protein Carbs, Fat	Comments
Jasmine Rice	0.25 cup (2.4oz)	160 cal	4g protein, 34g carbs, 2g fat	based on Lundberg's (uncooked Jasmine rice)
*Sweet and Sour Chicken	1 serving (4oz)	263.5 cal	37.5g protein, 12.5g carbs, 6.5g fat	Custom Workout Videos.com brand
*Sweet and Sour Sauce	1.5 servings (1.5oz)	89.5 cal	0g protein, 18g carbs, 1.5g fat	Custom Workout Videos.com brand

Men's Menu: Week Two

Breakfast	Serving Size	Calories	Grams Protein Carbs, Fat	Comments
Instant Oatmeal	1 pack (1.2oz)	130 cal	3g protein, 27g carbs, 2g fat	based on Quaker oatmeal (strawberry)
Blueberry Greek Yogurt	1 cup (6oz)	140 cal	14g protein, 20g carbs, 0g fat	based on no-fat Chobani brand yogurt
Banana	1 medium (4.2oz)	83 cal	1g protein, 21g carbs, 0.5g fat	based on an average organic brand

Snacks	Serving Size	Calories	Grams Protein Carbs, Fat	Comments
Granola Bar	0.5 package (1 bar)	80 cal	3g protein, 13g carbs, 2g fat	based on Nature Valley brand (apple crisp)
Creamy Peanut Butter	1 tbsp (0.6oz)	95 cal	4g protein, 3.5g carbs, 8g fat	based on Natural Creamy Jif

Lunch	Serving Size	Calories	Grams Protein Carbs, Fat	Comments
Pita Pocket Bread	1 pocket (2.4oz)	160 cal	6g protein, 32g carbs, 0g fat	based on Kangaroo Pita Pockets
Deli Meat Smoked Turkey or Roast Beef	1.5 servings (3oz)	90 cal	18g protein, 0g carbs, 4.5g fat	based on Applegate Farms deli meat
Sharp Cheddar or Swiss Cheese Slice	1 slice (1oz)	110 cal	7g protein, 0g carbs, 9g fat	based on Trader Joes sharp cheddar cheese
Butterhead Lettuce	2 slices (0.4oz)	<1cal	0g protein, <1g carbs, 0g fat	based on an average organic brand

Roma Tomatoes	4 slices (2.8oz)	14 cal	<1g protein, 3g carbs, 0g fat	based on an average organic brand
Yellow Mustard	1-2 tsp (0.2oz)	0 cal	0g protein, <1g carbs, 0g fat	based on French's classic yellow mustard

Snacks	Serving Size	Calories	Grams Protein Carbs, Fat	Comments
Deli Meat Smoked Turkey or Roast Beef	0.5 servings (1oz)	30 cal	6g protein, 0g carbs, 1.5g fat	based on Applegate Farms deli meat
Rosemary Olive Oil Crackers	6 crackers (1oz)	120 cal	3g protein, 20g carbs, 4g fat	based on Triscuit's brand
Sharp Cheddar or Swiss Cheese Slice	1 slice (1oz)	110 cal	7g protein, 0g carbs, 9g fat	based on Trader Joes sharp cheddar cheese
Sweet Bell Peppers	10 strips (1oz)	5 cal	0.5g protein, 1g carbs, 0g fat	based on an average organic brand (any color)

Dinner	Serving Size	Calories	Grams Protein Carbs, Fat	Comments
Jasmine Rice	0.33 cup (2.4oz)	240 cal	6g protein, 51g carbs, 3g fat	based on Lundberg's (uncooked Jasmine rice)
*Sweet and Sour Chicken	1 serving (4oz)	263.5 cal	37.5g protein, 12.5g carbs, 6.5g fat	Custom Workout Videos.com brand
*Sweet and Sour Sauce	1.5 servings (1.5oz)	89.5 cal	0g protein, 18g carbs, 1.5g fat	Custom Workout Videos.com brand

Your Second Cardio Plan

Modifications and Benefits

Benefits

Your second cardiovascular program is designed to make major improvements in your cardiorespiratory system by strengthening your heart and increasing your lung capacity.

Improving your heart strength and lung capacity is a major part of **The Six-Week Body Challenge**. If you're a heart attack survivor, or are prone to heart disease or have high blood pressure, you know the importance of strengthening your heart and lungs. According to the Center for Disease Control (CDC), high blood pressure and heart disease is the number one cause of death in the United States.

People of all ages and conditions can develop high blood pressure and heart disease, causing their heart to work harder than normal to pump out blood. This puts more force against the arterial walls, increasing blood pressure. In addition, if you have a diet that 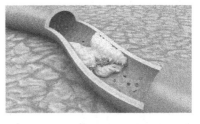 is high in fat coupled with a low level of cardiovascular fitness, it can lead to heart disease and may even potentially lead to cardiac arrest or a heart attack. This is especially true if you have high levels of bad cholesterol blocking your major arteries.

By increasing your intensity and improving cardiovascular condition, we can make your heart stronger and more efficient. Your heart will pump out more blood with less effort. This will decrease the force against your arteries, lower your blood pressure and make it easier for you to not only complete your circuit training programs but your other daily activities as well. All while losing weight!!!

Your Second Cardio Program

For your cardio program this week, let's go for a run. This is a great way to help build up your endurance and kick your calorie burning into high gear.

Make sure to alternate between walking for your warm-up and running for your cardio.

Warm Up (7-10 min) Begin by performing 7-10 minutes of light cardio by walking on the treadmill before you engage in your workout routine. Your heart rate should be between 100-120 bpm (beats per minute). This is about 50-55% of your maximum heart rate. This zone will be used to warm up your 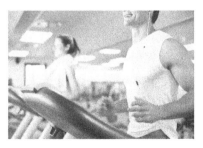 body and get you ready for your circuit training program.

Cardio: End of Program (10-15 min) Finish your program with 10-15 minutes of cardio by running on the treadmill once more. This is your cardio time, so get your heart rate up between 150-170 bpm.

This is roughly 65-75% of your maximum heart rate. This preferred training zone will make vast improvements to your cardiorespiratory system while still burning up to 50% of your calories as fat. During this program, you will only be able to comfortably speak small phrases, and you will be breathing much harder than when you were training on the upright bike. These physiological cues can reinforce when you're training at the right intensity. Push yourself hard this week. You deserve it!

Program Modifications

If you are not in good cardiovascular condition, you can do some light jogging on the treadmill with a slight incline instead of running. Either way, it will be your job to make sure that you are getting your heart rate up to match your training intensity from last week of 140-160 bpm. However, be sure to slow down if you get dizzy, lightheaded or are unable to catch your breath.

Also, if you don't have access to a treadmill, here are some suggestions:

1. Go to your local community center or YMCA. They should have a treadmill you can use along with some space and equipment you can use for your exercise routine afterward. (Community centers also tend to cost very little to use for the day and tend to have running tracks for use even if they don't have a treadmill.)

2. Go for a run or jog outside before your workout. If it is cold outside, you can jog or run in place at home as long as you work to get your heart rate up. No excuses!

Slimming Down! Workout Two

What to Know

Your second program is an important part of your exercise progression. The exercises in your second program are designed to accelerate your weight loss, stretch out your hips and low back, and strengthen the muscles surrounding your knees to improve structure and function.

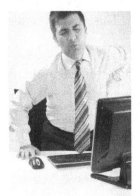

Sitting or leaning forward for long periods of time is a common source of hip and lower back pain. When you sit for long periods of time, the muscles that attach to your hips and your lower back shorten pulling your hips forward and causing your stomach to hang down. This condition, which is also known as having an Anterior Pelvic Tilt, will not only shorten your hips and lower back muscles (causing pain), but it will also make your midsection appear pudgy and weak.

To help with this problem, I've given you some exercises such as front and back squats to not only strengthen your legs, hamstrings and lower back, but to also stretch these muscles dynamically through a full range of motion. This will give your stomach a flatter appearance and restore the proper function and mobility in your hips and low back.

The exercises in this program will also start developing your quadriceps muscles (thigh muscles) as well as tightening up your glutes to give you a nice, firm butt. Developing your thigh muscles is extremely important because when you thighs are weak, you have a greater chance of injuring your knees. By strengthening your leg muscles during your workout, you can get your heart rate up faster and burn more calories. Also, as an added bonus to your second program, I added a lot of upper-body exercises to strengthen and tone your arms, shoulders, and back!

Slimming Down! Workout Two

Let's Get Started!!!

Slimming Down! Workout Two

Protocol and Order:

- ◆ **(Warm Up)** Walk on the treadmill for 7-10 minutes, keeping your heart rate between 100-120 bpm.

- ◆ **(Exercise)** Perform *two to three* circuits in order, keeping your heart rate between 140-160 bpm.

- ◆ **(Cardio)** Run for 10-15 minutes on the treadmill after your program with your heart rate between 150-170 bpm.

- ◆ **(Stretch)** Cool down using the stretches provided in this guide.

Duration: Week Two

Days per week: 2-3 (Leave 24 hours between sessions)

Exercise Reps: 10-12 or 12-15, depending on excercise

Load: Body weight or 30-40% 1 rep max

Circuits: 2-3

Rest interval: 15-30 seconds between exercises; 3-4 minutes between circuits

Equipment: Women: 12-15 lb body bar, two 5-8 lb dumbbells, and a 6 lb medicine ball

Men: 18-24 lb body bar, two 8-10 lb dumbbells, two 10-12 lb dumbbells, and an 8 lb medicine ball

Note: The last few reps on each exercise should be taxing. When you can comfortably perform the number of repetitions suggested, increase your weight.

get skinny!

Front Squat #1

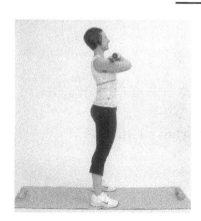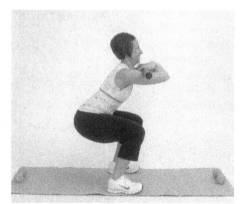

a. Start by standing upright with your feet slightly wider than shoulder-width apart. Grab the body bar first with your left hand and then with your right so your right arm is over your left. While holding on to the bar, lift your chest and raise your elbows until they're parallel to the floor. Let the bar rest on top of your shoulders.

b. Lower your body by bending at your knees while sticking your butt out until your knees and hips are parallel. Keep your chest up and at a 45° angle to your hips when squatting. This is to avoid any rounding in the back, which can cause you lower back pain.

c. While standing up, drive your hips forward until you can squeeze your butt cheeks together and your hips are aligned in a neutral position with your spine. Return and repeat. (Keep the bar horizontal throughout the exercise.)

Perform: 12-15 repetitions
Women: 12-15 lb body bar
Men: 18-24 lb body bar

Back Squat # 2

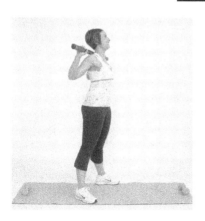 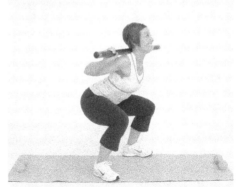

a. Stand upright with your feet slightly wider than shoulder-width apart. Tighten your upper back by pinching your shoulder blades together, and rest the bar on the muscles of your upper back, just below the bone at the top of your shoulder blades. Your hands should be shoulder-width apart with your palms out and your elbows back. This will protect your elbows from injuries.

b. Lower your body by bending at your knees while sticking your butt out until your knees and hips are parallel. Keep your chest up and at a 45° angle to your hips when squatting. (Keep the bar horizontal.)

c. While standing up, push up through your heels and drive your hips forward until you can squeeze your butt cheeks together. Your hips should be aligned in a neutral position with your spine when done. Return and repeat.

Perform: 12-15 repetitions
Women: 12-15 lb body bar
Men: 18-24 lb body bar

Upright Row # 3

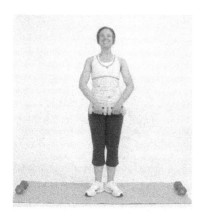 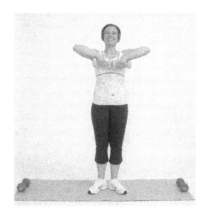

a. Stand with your back upright and feet together in a V-shape with your legs and glutes contracted.

b. Extend your arms downward with wrists and elbows in a straight line and palms pronated (facing toward your body).

c. Raise your weights by bending your elbows upward. Move the weights along your body until your elbows are at a 90° angle and parallel with the floor.

d. Hold and return the dumbbells down your body in the same way you brought them up. Repeat.

Special Instructions:

Keep your elbows elevated and above your wrists while you are lifting the weights.

Perform: 10-12 repetitions
Women: 5-8 lb dumbbells (each hand)
Men: 10-12 lb dumbbells (each hand)

Medicine Ball Slam # 4

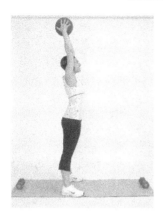 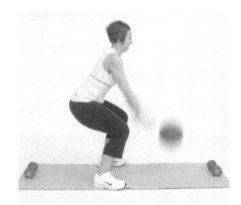

a. Stand with your feet slightly wider than shoulder-width apart and turn your toes out until your knees and hips are in a straight line.

b. Grab the medicine ball between your hands, pull it back behind your head, and hold it at arm's length overhead.

c. Forcefully throw the ball down on the ground as hard as possible while moving into a squat. (Keep your arms straight while slamming the ball on the ground.)

d. Catch the ball as it bounces up from the ground. Stand, return to starting position, and repeat.

Special Instructions:

This is a timed exercise. Complete all of your reps in 20-25 seconds.

Perform: 12-15 repetitions
Women: 6 lb medicine ball
Men: 8 lb medicine ball

Lateral Shoulder Raise to Stop Sign # 5

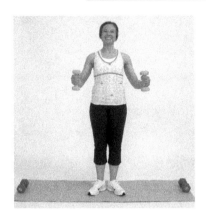 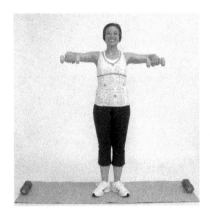

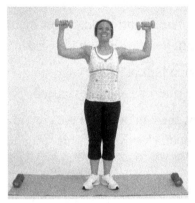

a. **(Part 1)** Stand with your back upright and feet together in a V-shape with legs and glutes contracted. Keep your back upright, shoulders relaxed and elbows bent.

b. Start with your elbows bent and in towards your sides, not touching. Elbows must be about 2-3 inches from your sides during the beginning and end of the exercise to fully engage the medial deltoid. This starting and ending position looks similar to a bench press.

c. Slowly raise the weights by lifting your elbows straight out to your sides until they are in line with your shoulders.

d. **(Part 2)** Look up, inhale, and slowly rotate your arms backward like a crossing guard raising a stop sign until your first resistance barrier.

e. Slowly rotate your arms back to the bench press position, and drop your elbows back down to your sides until they're 2-3 inches from your sides. Repeat.

Perform: 12-15 repetitions
Women: 5-8 lb dumbbells (each hand)
Men: 8-10 lb dumbbells (each hand)

Your Second Stretching Routine

Now that you're done with your workout, let's cool down!

What to Know

Your second exercise routine is designed to build the strength of your quadriceps muscles to help prevent knee injuries. It's also designed to maximize the development of your gluteal muscles to prevent lower back and hip pain.

Because the front and back squats in your second routine can make your quads, hips, and glutes tight, your second stretching routine is designed to help stretch these muscles out. I also added some neck and trap stretches to reduce neck tension and soreness after your workout.

Sitting Trap Stretch

- Sit on the ball and put your right arm be-tween your legs with your upper arm pressed against your thigh.

- Twist your torso, lifting your left arm up in the air until your shoulders are in line with one another, and look up.

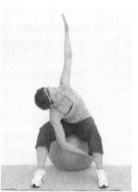

Stretching Benefits:

Tight middle back muscles can put pressure on your ribs and diaphragm. This can cause shortness of breath, pain that radiates to the front of your chest, and an inability to take a deep breath.

Perform: 2 sets of 1 repetition
Sides: Both
Hold stretch for 30 seconds.

Levator Scapulae Stretch

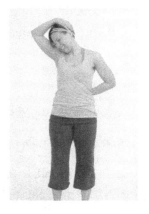

- Position your right arm behind your back if you are standing or grab under a chair if you are sitting.

- Tip your head toward your left shoulder and grab the back of your head with your left hand.

- Gently pull down on your head. Avoid lifting your shoulder while you are stretching.

Stretching Benefits:

Tight levator scapulae muscles can cause neck tension and pain, headaches, and shoulder stiffness.

Perform: 2 sets of 1 repetition
Sides: Both
Hold stretch for 30 seconds.

Side-Lying Quad Stretch

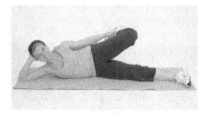

- Lie on one side, grab your ankle or foot, and bend your knee backward.

- Straighten your hip by pulling your ankle or foot backward, keeping your knee bent. Don't let your knee extend too far upward beyond your hip.

Stretching Benefits:

Tight quadriceps muscles can cause knee problems by changing the way your knee cap slides (patellar tracking) when extending your leg.

Perform: 2 sets of 1 repetition
Sides: Both
Hold stretch for 30 seconds.

Lying Piriformis Stretch

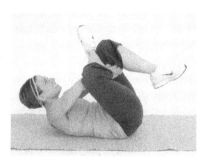

- Lie down on your back and cross your right leg over your left.

- Reach through your legs to grab your left leg and pull it towards your chest.

- Use your right elbow to push on your right knee until you feel the stretch in your gluteal muscle on the right side.

Stretching Benefits:

Tight piriformis muscles can put pressure on your sciatic nerves causing pain.

Perform: 2 sets of 1 repetition
Sides: Both
Hold stretch for 30 seconds.

Butterfly Stretch

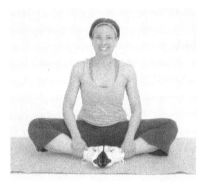

- Sit on the floor, bend both knees, and bring the soles of your feet together.

- Keep your back upright and slowly lean forward.

- Use your elbows and press your knees toward the floor until you feel a light stretch in your inner thighs.

Stretching Benefits:

Tight hip adductor muscles can cause your femur to become internally rotated. Since the knee joint will no longer be aligned properly, this can lead to knee pain (similar to tight quads).

Perform: 2 sets of 1 repetition
Hold stretch for 30 seconds.

get skinny!

Arm-Shoulder (Towel) Stretch

- Grab a hand towel and extend one hand down your back with your hand in line with your spine, pointing down.

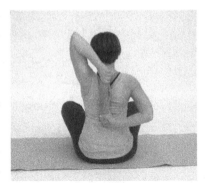

- Use the other hand to reach behind your back to grab the towel.

- Gently pull down on the towel, and then repeat by pulling up on the towel with the other hand.

Stretching Benefits:

Tight shoulders can cause your muscles to become weak, leading to shoulder dysfunction and pain.

Perform: 2 sets of 1 repetition
Sides: Both
Hold stretch for 30 seconds.

Chapter 3

overcoming comfort foods

His Voice of Reason

My name is Greg. I am 43 years old, and I live in Rhode Island. Recently, while sitting in the beautiful white sands of Second Beach in Newport, I remembered how much I hated being at the beach when I was overweight. I was so ashamed of my body, but no matter how bad I felt, I could never quite seem to bring myself to take action. That was until I turned 36 and developed two strong motivations to change my life: My health was beginning to deteriorate, and I desperately wanted to restore the pride that I once had in myself.

As a teenager, I grew up in the small suburb town of East Greenwich, Rhode Island where I was very active in sports and in my school's theater department. After all, I had to be physically active to participate in all of my extracurricular activities as well as to impress the girls at school.

But a lot of that began to change when I went to college. I was a confident, good-looking kid while at college, but I began to lose my hair. Ugh—what a traumatic experience! (It was really tramautic for my roommates too, especially because I was constantly clogging our shower drain!) I was too young to go bald. I tried every shampoo, lotion, and spray-on remedy that I could get my hands on, but nothing seemed to work. Then, suddenly, my hair started to grow back! But instead of it being on my head, it was all over my back.

It got so bad, in fact, that when swimming with a friend, he jokingly asked me to take my sweater off. It may have been funny if he was talking about an actual sweater and not my back hair. This was how my sense of self worth first started to deteiorate.

While in college, I remember reading an interview with Alicia Silverstone, my favorite actress from the movie "Clueless." In the inverview, she listed balding men with hairy backs as one of her biggest turnoffs. I figured that Silverstone's opinion was how most women viewed men with hariy backs. I remember feeling very self-conscious and unattractive after reading that article.

Fortunately, I didn't let that stop me from talking to the girls, nor did it prevent me from getting married. But after I graduated college, my sense of self worth took another hit when I found myself putting in long hours at work to advance my career. Although I managed to maintain my weight, I noticed my metabolism was starting to change. My body began to take longer to recover after my weekend activities, and my cholesterol levels were rising with each annual checkup.

When I was 32, my family began to grow with the birth of our first child, and life was keeping me busier than ever. To continually advance myself at my career, I had to work extremely long days, and when I came home, I needed to spend my free time helping my wife take care of our children. In fact, the only "me time" that I had was late at night, in front of the TV, where I would eat comfort food to get rid of the stress. I started gorging myself night after night on unhealthy snacks to make me feel better, and even though it worked, my "couch potato" relaxation routine continued to impact my health and my metabolism, making things worse.

As a consequence of my unhealthy eating habits, I ballooned from 180 pounds as a teenager, to over 200 pounds in my twenties, until I finally reached well over 240 pounds at the age of 36.

After my annual checkup that year, my doctor recommended that I lose weight after he once again confirmed that I had high-blood pressure and a cholesterol level of 240. He told me that my prognosis was typical for a hard-working father in his thirties, but that I had to take some action before things got worse. If I didn't, he said, I was headed for a lifetime of stress, medications, and heart problems. I knew that I had wanted to lose weight so many times before, but it wasn't that easy. I had other self-confidence issues that I needed to address first, namely my body hair.

When I was overweight, I would often think, *Why am I so unhappy? Is it because I am overweight, or is it because I am cursed with such a hairy back? And why should I lose weight? I'm still going to be hairy!* It really affected my self image, and I often wondered if being hairy and overweight was the main reason so many men have a tough time getting into shape. After all, even if they get into shape, they are still going to be hairy and unsightly.

I didn't know what to do, but I knew that I had to stop worrying about what other people thought of me if I was going to change. So, I decided to pursue laser hair treatments for my body. But even after the hair problem was solved, I found that I still didn't feel comfortable with taking my shirt off at the beach. Not with my belly.

I was still really unhappy with how I looked, and I felt even worse after reading an article that listed common body blunders that men make. The article metioned that one of things women find most unattractive is a man with a "beer belly." The article also mentioned that if you think your significant other will love you no matter what you look like, you are probably wrong. This really helped shed light on a big double standard that I was carrying around: I had expected my wife to maintain her beauty while I had just let myself go.

I knew then and there that if I was going to get in shape, I would need an easy plan that would fit my busy schedule. The plan also had to be simple because I was such a comfort eater. It was so much easier for me to just relax at the end of the night with my junk food than it was to watch what I was eating, especially when I'd had a rough day at work.

Fortunately, I remembered that back in my high school days, when I was most fit, I did not eat much fat or sugar, and I was a lot more physically active with sports and drama. I decided to get over my comfort eating and take things seriously. I had to do this for my wife, for my family, and to reclaim my feelings of pride and self worth.

I started to eat more frequently throughout the day, and I started by cutting back on sugar intake. At first, I found this difficult because I either didn't feel full or I didn't like the way that low-sugar foods tasted. I began experimenting with healthier alternatives to increase my fiber and protein intake while reducing my fat calories and sugar. I began looking for healthier alternatives for the comfort foods that I loved to eat to make it easier for me to stick with my diet, and I implemented simple exercises into my weekly routine.

And I was shocked. It was working! I lost thirty pounds within the first two months of implementing my new routine. My cholesterol dropped to 190, and a few months after that, I had lost another twenty pounds. My body also started to get really toned from the weekly exercises.

● ● ● ● ● ● ● ● ● ● ●
*Carbohydrate fun fact: Your brain can only use sugar for energy.
● ● ● ● ● ● ● ● ● ● ●

I recently turned 43. I have maintained a healthy weight for over seven years, and I now weigh similar to what I did in high school: 185 pounds. The best part about my new body is that I can proudly remove my shirt at the beach. My weight-loss plan was so successful that it was published as a diet book in 2009 called *The Couch Potato Diet.*

(www.**TheCouchPotatoDiet**.com)

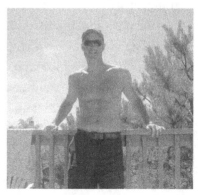

This is actually how I met Scott. He designed exercise routines not only for me and my family, but also for one of my books. I have been able to implement his workouts into my weekly routines, and they have helped me to stay fit and strong. And I know you can do it too!

No matter how busy you are or how good it feels to eat when things aren't working out, trust me, food isn't the answer. Make small changes and remember to stay strong. Today can be your first step to a better future!

Our Need for Carbs

Understanding Carbohydrates and Why We Crave This Invigorating Nutrient.

Carbohydrates

Everyone has heard a little something about carbs and either love them or hate them. They are fun, controversial and misunderstood!

Understanding this nutrient is essential to your success because carbohydrates are an important part of **The Six-Week Body Challenge.** Carbohydrates or saccharides play a critical role in your diet by providing you with the energy necessary to power every function in your body. They also trigger your satiety mechanism, making you feel full at the end of a meal. Similarly, going too long without carbohydrates will cause you to feel weak, sluggish, dizzy, and light-headed.

Carbohydrates are extremely useful because they provide the energy necessary for your body to function. However, if you consume too many carbs, your body will store the excess as fat instead of burning it for energy. So, when it comes to losing weight, should you eat carbs or stay away from them all together?

Let's take a look at what carbohydrates are and what they do. This will help you understand my carbohydrate recommendations for your **Six-Week Body Challenge**.

The Break Down

When carbohydrates are broken down by your body, they are converted into glucose or blood sugar, and with the help of insulin, they provide the energy your cells need to function. Insulin is released by the pancreas when blood sugar levels rise and helps your body's cells metabolize the sugar in your bloodstream. It also helps your body store energy (sugar) in your muscle tissue and liver for later use. These are called glycogen stores.

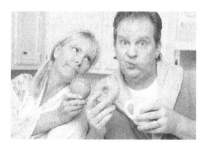

The more physically active you are, the more carbohydrates you'll need for energy. However, not all carbs are created equal. There are two types of carbohydrates: simple and complex. When choosing the types of carbohydrates to add into your diet, especially now that you are increasing your activity level, I recommend adding more complex carbs and cutting down on your intake of simple carbs. Complex carbs give you longer more sustained energy and are better for your health.

1. *Simple Carbohydrates* contain one or two sugar molecules (mono or disaccharide) and are easily absorbed into the bloodstream, offering you immediate but short-term energy. Simple carbs usually don't contain any vitamins, minerals or fiber. They are basically empty calories, and consuming them makes it difficult to lose weight.

2. *Complex Carbohydrates* have larger chains of sugars (polysaccharides or starches) and take longer to be broken down before being absorbed into your bloodstream to be utilized for energy. This slower breakdown helps stabilize your blood sugar levels, helping to curb your appetite and giving you more sustained energy throughout the day. Complex carbs also offer a wide variety of vitamins, minerals and fiber to help your body run efficiently.

Carbs are Important for Exercise

When you exercise, your body needs different energy from different sources, which are dependent on the type of exercise routine you are doing. **The Six-Week Body Challenge** uses circuit training, which is a moderate intensity exercise requiring sugar for energy. Carbohydrates (converted to glucose) are important for this type of workout since they can be metabolized by your body faster than fat and protein.

Fat and protein are used for energy during low intensity activities like sitting, walking or biking. During low intensity exercises, the body goes through a process called "glucose sparing" and does not use its sugar reserves or glycogen stores for energy. The body burns both fat and protein for energy instead of sugar, but the energy output is low and takes a long time to metabolize. As the intensity of your exercise increases, so does your need for sugar.

Sugar is metabolized by the body more rapidly than fat or protein. Because of this, the body needs more carbs as the intensity rises. The body can also metabolize the sugar reserves (glycogen stores) in your liver for energy as your need for sugar increases. For **The Six-Week Body Challenge**, you will need these sugar stores to help you complete your exercise routines.

If you do not have a moderate amount of carbohydrates in your system, your body will hit nervous system fatigue. Since your nervous system is only powered by glucose, when you run low on carbohydrates, your nervous system starts to tire. This makes the communication signals that travel from your nervous system to your body become slower and decline in strength, making it difficult for you to finish your exercise routine.

Since your body needs sugar when you're exercising at higher intensities, I want you to consume a moderate amount of carbohydrates each day to help keep your glycogen stores full. This will not only help you with your exercise routines, but it will also allow you to burn more fat and total calories by allowing you to exercise at a higher intensity.

Over-Consumption (Blood Sugar Imbalance)

Calculating the amount of carbohydrates you need to consume each day should be based on how many calories you need to eat and on how physically active you are. This will allow you to efficiently use the energy you are consuming on a daily basis and keep your glycogen stores full (the sugar reserves in the liver and muscle tissue). If you are 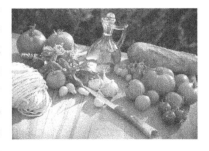 consuming more carbohydrates than your body can use, your glycogen stores will never become depleted, and your body will store the rest of the sugar as fat in your body. This happens in a rather simple process:

1. Carbohydrates break down into glucose to be used for energy causing blood sugar levels to rise.

2. When blood sugar levels rise, insulin is released into your bloodstream to help your cells metabolize the sugar for energy. (This process lowers your blood sugar levels.)

3. Some of the extra sugar is stored in your muscle tissue and liver (glycogen stores) for later use.

4. Any excess sugar that wasn't used or stored for energy, especially over long periods of time, will be stored as fat in your body.

So, how many carbohydrates do you need to consume to have an adequate amount of energy without storing the excess as body fat?

How Many Carbohydrates Do You Need?

On a daily basis, the average person needs between 40% and 65% of his or her total calories from carbohydrates. Where you fall in this range depends on how physically active you are. For the purposes of this body challenge, I designed your menus so that 50% of your total calories come from carbohydrates.

● ● ● ● ● ● ● ● ● ● ●

Carb Activity Range:
40-45%: sedentary
to low activity
45-55%: moderately active
55-65%: highly active

● ● ● ● ● ● ● ● ● ● ●

For Men: Each week, your daily menu contains a total of 1,800 calories with 50% of those calories coming from carbohydrates. This means that you're consuming a total of 900 calories of carbs each and every day. From there, it is very easy to convert that number into grams. There are four calories for every gram of carbohydrates that you eat (just like protein), so you simply divide 900 calories by four, which works out to 250 grams of carbs per day.

For Women: Each week, your daily menu contains a total of 1,400 calories, and because you are also consuming 50% of your total calories from carbohydrates, your total daily intake of carbs needs to equal 700 calories. To convert this into grams, we'll figure it out the same way that we did for the men: dividing your total intake of 700 calories by four. This means that you need to consume 175 grams of carbohydrates each day to give your body the energy it needs to complete your workouts and other daily activities.

Choose Your Carbs Wisely

Nutrition experts (myself included) recommend getting carbohydrates from the following sources:

- **Starchy Vegetables:** Dark leafy green leaf lettuces along with asparagus, celery, rhubarb, broccoli, cauliflower, turnips and carrots are excellent sources of complex carbohydrates. Fruit vegetables such as avocado, tomato, cucumber, zucchini, and eggplant are also wonderful sources of starchy vegetables. Vegetables are important for your diet because they contain lots of vitamins, minerals and fiber. Vitamins and minerals repair wear and tear to the body, and fiber helps prevent constipation.

- **Beans (Legumes):** Beans or legumes include lentils, garbanzo, pinto, kidney, black and white beans. Lima beans and other dried beans, such as black-eyed peas, are also a great choice. Beans are starchy and are loaded with fiber, which helps you feel full and avoid constipation. To help avoid the gassy side effects of some beans, soak and boil your beans before eating.

- **Peas and Corn:** Peas and corn are also great sources of complex carbohydrates. Try adding white and yellow corn into your diet along with peas like split green, yellow, snap and snow peas.

- **Whole grains:** Whole grains contain a lot of fiber, plenty of Vitamin B and other minerals like iron, which help carry oxygen in your blood. This is very helpful when exercising and for women during menstruation.

There are, however, carbs that are not good for your body. I recommend staying away from sugars such as table sugar, corn syrup, dextrose, maltose, lactose, and sucrose. Also, limit your consumption of honey, candy, soda pop, packaged cereals, baked goods, and breads and pastas made with white flour.

Your Third Menu

Menu Benefits (Reducing Free Radical Damage)

This week's menu gives you just the right amount of carbohydrate energy you need to exercise at a more intense pace, allowing you to lose weight faster and feel great. As you work out at this pace, however, you'll breathe more deeply and consume more oxygen, which can lead to a faster oxidation of your body's cells and free radical damage.

To help you counteract these affects, this week's menu is packed full of farm-fresh fruits and vegetables, mouthwatering berries, delectable whole grains and savory lean meats to give your body all of the antioxidants it needs to repair free radical damage. This menu also includes a satisfying fried rice dish that is sure to put a smile on your face!

Notes on This Week's Menu

Need a change in your routine? It's okay to change the order of your meals as long as you make sure to stay with the same serving and portion sizes. Also, remember to record your weight and your measurements again at the beginning of the week and to take some follow-up pictures.

Your breakfast this week is intended to be a deliciously satisfying, antioxidant-filled raspberry yogurt parfait. This should be a quick and easy meal for you to make, especially if you are on the go in the mornings. Enjoy!

Special Entrée of the Week

Fried Rice gives you the same great taste of takeout without the hassle of going out. This recipe can also be made with fresh chunks of farm- raised chicken instead of egg whites for a satisfying and delicious chicken fried rice dish.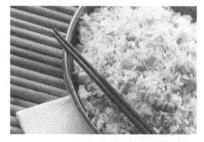

This recipe is available for only $0.99 at:
CustomWorkoutVideos.com/catalog/index.php

Women's Menu: Week Three

Breakfast	Serving Size	Calories	Grams Protein Carbs, Fat	Comments
Blueberry Greek Yogurt	1 cup (6oz)	140 cal	14g protein, 20g carbs, 0g fat	based on no-fat Chobani brand yogurt
Raspberries	0.5 cup (2.2oz)	32 cal	1g protein, 7g carbs, 0.5g fat	based on an average organic brand
Granola Bar	0.5 package (1 bar)	80 cal	3g protein, 13g carbs, 2g fat	based on Nature Valley brand (apple crisp)

Snacks	Serving Size	Calories	Grams Protein Carbs, Fat	Comments
Cottage Cheese	0.5 cup (3.9oz)	112 cal	14g protein, 5g carbs, 5g fat	based on Organic Valley brand
Dried Raisins	0.5 small box (0.5oz)	46 cal	0.5g protein, 11g carbs, 0g fat	based on Sun-Maid raisins
Cinnamon (to taste) and Agave Nectar	1 tbsp (1oz)	60 cal	0g protein, 16g carbs, 0g fat	based on Madhava brand agave nectar

Lunch	Serving Size	Calories	Grams Protein Carbs, Fat	Comments
Pita Pocket Bread	0.5 pocket (2.4oz)	80 cal	3g protein, 16g carbs, 0g fat	based on Kangaroo Pita Pockets
Deli Meat Smoked Turkey or Roast Beef	1.5 servings (3oz)	90 cal	18g protein, 0g carbs, 4.5g fat	based on Applegate Farms deli meat
Sharp Cheddar or Swiss Cheese Slice	1 slice (1oz)	110 cal	7g protein, 0g carbs, 9g fat	based on Trader Joes sharp cheddar cheese

Butterhead Lettuce	2 slices (0.4oz)	<1cal	0g protein, <1g carbs, 0g fat	based on an average organic brand
Roma Tomatoes	4 slices (2.8oz)	14 cal	<1g protein, 3g carbs, 0g fat	based on an average organic brand
Yellow Mustard	1-2 tsp (0.2oz)	0 cal	0g protein, <1g carbs, 0g fat	based on French's classic yellow mustard

Snacks	Serving Size	Calories	Grams Protein Carbs, Fat	Comments
Chocolate Fudge Brownie	1 bar	90 cal	1g protein, 18g carbs, 3g fat	based on Fiber One Brand
Banana	1 medium (4.2oz)	120 cal	1g protein, 27g carbs, 0.5g fat	based on an average organic brand

Dinner	Serving Size	Calories	Grams Protein Carbs, Fat	Comments
*Fried Rice	1 serving (1 cup)	320 cal	9g protein, 50g carbs, 10g fat	Custom Workout Videos.com brand
Liquid Egg Whites	2 servings (0.5 cup)	50 cal	10g protein, 2g carbs, 0g fat	based on Organic Valley liquid egg whites

Men's Menu: Week Three

Breakfast	Serving Size	Calories	Grams Protein Carbs, Fat	Comments
Blueberry Greek Yogurt	1 cup (6oz)	140 cal	14g protein, 20g carbs, 0g fat	based on no-fat Chobani brand yogurt
Raspberries	0.5 cup (2.2oz)	32 cal	1g protein, 7g carbs, 0.5g fat	based on an average organic brand
Granola Bar	0.5 package (1 bar)	80 cal	3g protein, 13g carbs, 2g fat	based on Nature Valley brand (apple crisp)

Snacks	Serving Size	Calories	Grams Protein Carbs, Fat	Comments
Cottage Cheese	1 cup (7.8oz)	224 cal	28g protein, 10g carbs, 10g fat	based on Organic Valley brand
Dried Raisins	0.5 small box (0.5oz)	46 cal	0.5g protein, 11g carbs, 0g fat	based on Sun-Maid raisins
Cinnamon (to taste) and Agave Nectar	1 tbsp (1oz)	60 cal	0g protein, 16g carbs, 0g fat	based on Madhava brand agave nectar

Lunch	Serving Size	Calories	Grams Protein Carbs, Fat	Comments
Pita Pocket Bread	1 pocket (2.4oz)	160 cal	6g protein, 32g carbs, 0g fat	based on Kangaroo Pita Pockets
Deli Meat Smoked Turkey or Roast Beef	1.5 servings (3oz)	90 cal	18g protein, 0g carbs, 4.5g fat	based on Applegate Farms deli meat
Sharp Cheddar or Swiss Cheese Slice	1 slice (1oz)	110 cal	7g protein, 0g carbs, 9g fat	based on Trader Joes sharp cheddar cheese

Butterhead Lettuce	2 slices (0.4oz)	<1cal	0g protein, <1g carbs, 0g fat	based on an average organic brand
Roma Tomatoes	4 slices (2.8oz)	14 cal	<1g protein, 3g carbs, 0g fat	based on an average organic brand
Yellow Mustard	1-2 tsp (0.2oz)	0 cal	0g protein, <1g carbs, 0g fat	based on French's classic yellow mustard

Snacks	Serving Size	Calories	Grams Protein Carbs, Fat	Comments
Chocolate Fudge Brownie	1 bar	90 cal	1g protein, 18g carbs, 3g fat	based on Fiber One Brand
Banana	1 large (4.8oz)	136 cal	1.5g protein, 31g carbs, 0.5g fat	based on an average organic brand

Dinner	Serving Size	Calories	Grams Protein Carbs, Fat	Comments
*Fried Rice	1.5 servings (1 cup)	480 cal	13.5g protein, 75g carbs, 15g fat	Custom Workout Videos.com brand
Liquid Egg White	2.5 servings (0.75 cup)	75 cal	15g protein, 3g carbs, 0g fat	based on Organic Valley liquid egg whites

Your Third Cardio Plan

Modifications and Benefits

The Benefits

Your third cardiorespiratory program is designed to increase the stroke volume of your heart, making your heart efficient at pumping out blood with every beat. This will help get more oxygen to your vital systems quicker and prevent cardiovascular and muscular fatigue.

Cardiovascular conditioning is an extremely important component to **The Six-Week Body Challenge** because when your level of cardiovascular conditioning is low, your stroke volume will be low. This will make it difficult to complete your circuit training programs successfully since you'll be lacking the oxygen your muscles need. Having a poor stroke volume will also cause your heart and lungs to work hard even during simple chores and activities like carrying groceries, going for a walk, or going up and down a flight of stairs.

● ● ● ● ● ● ● ● ● ● ●
*Cardio Fun Fact: Men and women who are in better cardiovascular shape have lower resting heart rates.
● ● ● ● ● ● ● ● ● ● ●

By increasing your stroke volume, we can increase the strength and efficiency of your heart. Your body will pump out more blood and oxygen with every beat, reducing the number of times it needs to beat every minute. Increasing your stroke volume will be especially helpful as we increase the intensity of your cardio program. This program will help prepare your heart and lungs for the increase!

Your Third Cardio Program

Your circuit training program this week involves a lot of multi-planar motions designed to build your arm strength and blast your core. To make sure that both your upper and lower body are ready for action, let's tear it up by using the elliptical cross-trainer machine.

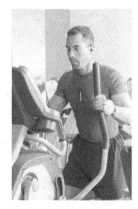

Warm Up (7-10 min) Warm up by performing 7-10 minutes of light cardio on the elliptical before you engage in your workout routine. I want your heart rate to be between 100-120 bpm. This training zone is designed to properly warm-up your body by oxygenating your muscles for activity and is about 50-55% of your maximum heart rate.

Cardio: End of Program (10-15 min) Perform 10-15 minutes of cardio on the elliptical cross-trainer after your program. This is your time to get your cardio on, so make sure to push yourself hard and get your heart rate up to be between 150-170 bpm.

This training zone is closer to 65-75% of your maximum heart rate, and you will only be able to comfortably speak small phrases when exercising at this intensity. You'll be breathing much harder than when you were training on the upright bike, and the level of intensity will feel similar to your running program. Use these physiological cues to reinforce when you are training within the right zone. The best part is that you'll still burn up to 50% of your calories from fat in this zone!

Next week, you'll be on the elliptical machine again, but I will be raising the intensity level to continue your momentum and accelerate your weight loss potential. Make sure to push yourself throughout the entire week so you'll be ready. I know you can do it!

Program Modifications

Your level of cardiovascular conditioning should be improving, but you may still need some modifications. If you do, you can alternate your heart rate on the elliptical cross-trainer between the higher training zone (150-170bpm) and the lower training zone from last week (140-160bpm) until your time is finished. Alternate the intensities by going for one minute at the higher intensity and then for two minutes at the lower intensity until you're done. Make sure to slow down if you get dizzy, lightheaded or are unable to catch your breath.

Also, if you don't have access to an elliptical, here are some suggestions:

1. Go to your local community center or YMCA. They should have a cross-trainer you can use along with some space and exercise equipment you can use for your exercise routine afterward.

2. If it's warm outside, go for a run or jog before your workout. If it's cold outside, buy a jump rope and do your cardio at home. Make sure to push yourself hard... no excuses!

Go For It! Workout Three

What to Know

In recent years, abdominal training and core training have come to mean the same thing, even though they're not. Your core consists of more than just your abdominal muscles. It includes the muscles that stabilize your spine, torso, and pelvis (hips and glutes) against gravity, creating a solid base of support. Your core muscles allow you to move your body freely about in any direction.

Traditional abdominal and core training have become synonymous with exercises like floor crunches and sit-ups. While these exercises can help you get a flatter stomach (with plenty of repetition), they are specifically designed to target your abs and not your core since they limit your body's range of motion during the exercise.

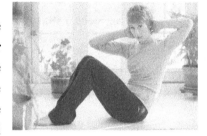

When you target any particular muscle group too much, you can create a muscular imbalance. This happens when one muscle group is stronger than its opposing muscle group—for example, the muscles in the front and the back of your torso (chest and back). While this may not sound serious, it could lead to a wide variety of problems including poor posture, sore muscles, and injury to your body's musculoskeletal system.

Because I want your **Six-Week Body Challenge** to be all about improving your quality of life, your third program is designed to take a nontraditional approach to core training. This means simultaneously strengthening your torso, hips, and back as one solid unit.

To help you do this, your third program includes a lot of multi-directional, multi-joint exercises like the Overhead Asymmetrical Squat and the Bicep Curl to Press. These different exercises will challenge your core muscles in unison to create rock-hard abs. They will also create a greater weight loss potential for you by increasing your heart rate and oxygen consumption during your workout. Plus, all of the exercises in your third program will help improve your body's flexibility and stability while simultaneously converting strength gained into usable power for reflex motion and other daily activities!

Go For It! Workout Three

Let's Get Started!!!

Go For It! Workout Three

Protocol and Order:

- **(Warm Up)** Perform 7-10 minutes of cardio on the elliptical cross-trainer before you start your routine, keeping your heart rate between 100-120 bpm.

- **(Exercise)** Perform *three to four* circuits in order, keeping your heart rate between 150-170 bpm.

- **(Cardio)** Perform 10-15 minutes on the elliptical after your program with your heart rate between 150-170 bpm.

- **(Stretch)** Cool down using the stretches in this guide.

Duration: Week Three

Days per week: 2-3 (Leave 24 hours between sessions)

Exercise Reps: 10-12

Load: Body weight or 55-65% 1 rep max

Circuits: 3-4

Rest interval: 15-30 seconds between exercises; 4-5 minutes between circuits

Equipment: Women: 18-24 lb body bar, two 5-8 lb dumbbells, and two 8-10 lb dumbbells

Men: 24-30 lb body bar, two 8-10 lb dumbbells, two 10-12 lb dumbbells, and two 12-15 lb dumbbells

Note: The last few reps on each exercise should be taxing. When you can comfortably perform the number of repetitions suggested, increase your weight.

Front Squat # 1

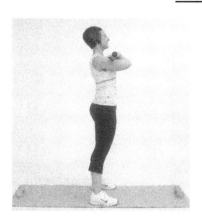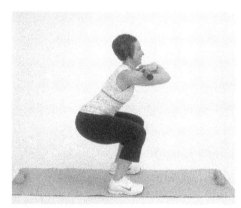

a. Stand upright with your feet slightly wider than shoulder-width apart. Grab the body bar first with your left hand and then with your right so your right arm is over your left. While holding onto the bar, lift your chest up and raise your elbows until they're parallel to the floor. Let the bar rest on top of your shoulders.

b. Lower your body by bending at your knees while sticking your butt out, and lower your body until your knees and hips are parallel. Keep your chest up and at a 45° angle to your hips when squatting.

c. While standing up, drive your hips forward until you can squeeze your butt cheeks together and your hips are aligned in a neutral position with your spine. Return and repeat. (Keep the bar horizontal throughout the exercise.)

Perform: 10-12 repetitions
Women: 18-24 lb body bar
Men: 24-30 lb body bar

Overhead Asymmetrical Squat # 2

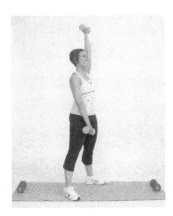 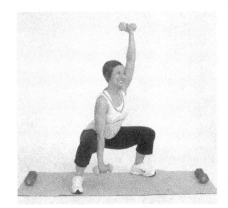

a. **(Part 1)** Stand with your feet slightly wider than shoulder-width apart and turn your toes out so your hips and knees are in a straight line. Grab two dumbbells and drop one arm/dumbbell between your legs. Lift your chest up and raise the other dumbbell straight up overhead with your palm facing outward.

b. **(Part 2)** Lower your body by bending at your knees while sticking your butt out, and continue squatting until your knees and hips are parallel. When squatting, keep your chest up and at a 45° angle to your hips while keeping the one dumbbell up overhead. Use your back, legs and core muscles to stabilize your body's position throughout the movement to avoid any rounding in your back.

c. **(Part 3)** While standing up, drive your hips forward until you can squeeze your butt cheeks together and until your hips and spine are in a neutral position. Complete all of your repetitions before switching sides and arms.

Perform: 10-12 repetitions
Women: 5-8 lb dumbbells (each hand)
Men: 10-12 lb dumbbells (each hand)

Bent-Over Flye (Rear Delt Raise) # 3

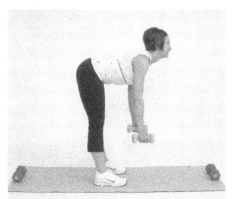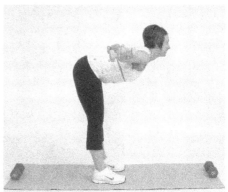

a. Grab the dumbbells with palms facing each other. Stand with your feet shoulder-width apart. Bend forward at the waist until your torso is parallel to the floor, and extend your arms and the dumbbells downward.

b. Fully straighten your legs by sticking your butt up and out while driving up through your heels. Lift your chest up, and keep your torso parallel to the floor to prevent strain to your lower back. If your hamstrings are too tight to fully straighten, it's okay to keep your knees slightly bent.

c. With your torso forward and stationary, exhale and lift the dumbbells straight to your sides until both arms are parallel to the floor with a slight bend in your elbows. Avoid swinging your torso or bringing your arms back instead of to your sides. Return and repeat.

Perform: 10-12 repetitions
Women: 5-8 lb dumbbells (each hand)
Men: 8-10 lb dumbbells (each hand)

Bicep Curl to Press # 4

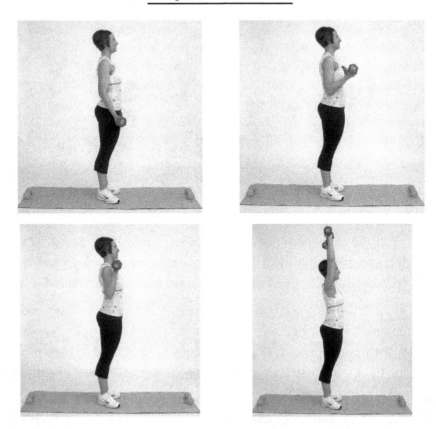

a. **(Part 1)** Hold a dumbbell in each hand with a soft grip, weights at your sides and palms facing upward.

b. Stand with your back upright and feet together in a V-shape with your legs and glutes contracted. Keep your back upright, shoulders relaxed and your elbows in.

c. Slowly raise the weights by bending your elbows inward until your knuckles are 3-4 inches away from your shoulders, and turn your palms facing outward.

d. **(Part 2)** Look up and inhale while pressing to keep your spine straight. Stop when your arms are extended straight overhead. Keep your wrists, shoulders and elbows in a straight line.

e. Exhale and slowly lower the weights back to the starting position in the same way you pressed up. Repeat.

Perform: 10-12 repetitions
Women: 8-10 lb dumbbells (each hand)
Men: 12-15 lb dumbbells (each hand)

Lateral Shoulder Raise to Stop Sign # 5

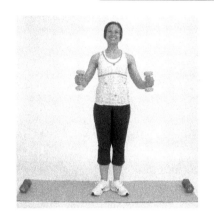
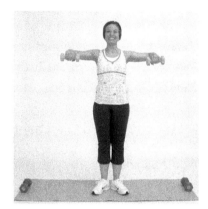
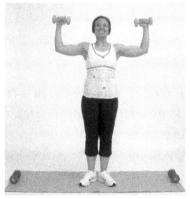

a. **(Part 1)** Stand with your back upright and feet together in a V-shape with legs and glutes contracted. Keep your back upright, shoulders relaxed and elbows bent.

b. Start with your elbows bent and in towards your sides, not touching. Your elbows must be about 2-3 inches from your sides during the beginning and end of the exercise to fully engage the medial deltoid. This starting and ending position looks similar to a bench press.

c. Slowly raise the weights by lifting your elbows straight out to your sides until they are in line with your shoulders.

d. **(Part 2)** Look up, inhale, and slowly rotate your arms backward like a crossing guard raising a stop sign until your first resistance barrier (looking up helps to avoid arching your back).

e. Exhale, slowly rotate your arms back to your bench press position, and drop your elbows back down to your sides until they are 2-3 inches from your sides. Repeat.

Perform: 10-12 repetitions
Women: 8-10 lb dumbbells (each hand)
Men: 10-12 lb dumbbells (each hand)

Your Third Stretching Routine

Now that you're done with your workout, let's cool down!

What to Know

Your third exercise routine is designed to strengthen your core muscles as well as your arms by using a lot of multi-planar, multi-joint exercises like the Overhead Asymmetrical Squat.

Your third stretching routine will help stretch the muscles in your neck, shoulders, and mid-back to alleviate any tension that was caused by the exercises in your workout program. It is also designed to loosen the muscles in your lower back to prevent any post-workout discomfort and soreness.

Scalene Neck Stretch

- Grab your left arm behind your back with your right hand and pull down.

- Look straight ahead and lean your head to your right side like you're trying to touch your ear to your shoulder.

- Avoid lifting your shoulder while stretching.

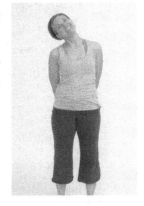

Stretching Benefits:

Tight scalene muscles are a common source of headaches, and tight scalene muscles can refer pain to the front of your chest causing false angina.

Perform: 2 sets of 1 repetition
Sides: Both
Hold stretch for 30 seconds.

Levator Scapulae Stretch

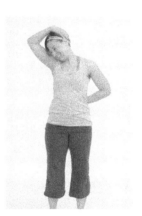

- Position your right arm behind your back if you're standing, or grab under a chair if you're sitting.

- Tip your head toward your left shoulder and grab the back of your head with your left hand.

- Gently pull down on your head without lifting your shoulder.

Stretching Benefits:

Tight levator scapulae muscles can make your neck so tight that it becomes difficult to turn your neck because of the tension and pain.

Perform: 2 sets of 1 repetition
Sides: Both
Hold stretch for 30 seconds.

Kneeling Hip Flexor Stretch

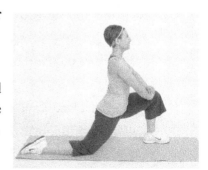

- Kneel down on one knee with your other leg out in front.

- Place your hands on your knees.

- Lean forward, keeping your chest and back upright until you can feel the stretch in the inside of your back leg.

Stretching Benefits:

Tight hip flexor muscles are a major source of hip and lower back pain when they rotate your hips out of alignment.

Perform: 2 sets of 1 repetition
Sides: Both
Hold stretch for 30 seconds.

Pigeon Pose (Glute) Stretch

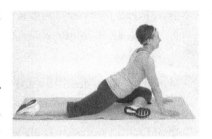

- Start on your hands and knees. Bend one leg out in front of you on the floor.

- Place the other leg straight behind you.

- Use your arms to slowly push your torso upright until you feel the stretch in the gluteal side of your bent leg.

Stretching Benefits:

The gluteal muscles maintain the mobility of your pelvis and sacrum. If they are tight, you'll have lower back and hip pain.

Perform: 2 sets of 1 repetition
Sides: Both
Hold stretch for 30 seconds.

Standing Side Stretch

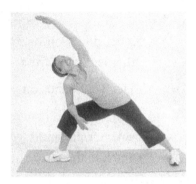

- Stand with your legs wide apart with your right leg out in front.

- Point your right toes straight forward and left toes out until both feet make a T-shape.

- Twist and place your right elbow on your thigh, straighten your left arm up, and stretch toward the opposite wall.

Stretching Benefits:

Tight latissimus dorsi muscles are a source of chronic shoulder and back pain.

Perform: 2 sets of 1 repetition
Sides: Both
Hold stretch for 30 seconds.

Sitting Trap Stretch

- Sit on the ball and put your right arm between your legs with your upper arm pressed against your thigh.

- Twist your torso, lift your left arm up in the air until your shoulders are in line with one another, and look up.

Stretching Benefits:

The muscles of your mid back attach to your vertebrae, and tight mid-back muscles can pull your vertebrae out of alignment, causing joint pain and dysfunction.

Perform: 2 sets of 1 repetition
Sides: Both
Hold stretch for 30 seconds.

the frog prince

Claiming His True Self

Children have special growth platelets and epiphyseal unions that are located at the end of each of their bones. They are soft tissues, designed to help the bones stretch and grow as the child ages. However, they are so fragile that an injury that would cause only a simple joint sprain in an adult could cause a growth platelet fracture in a child. And if treated improperly, these kinds of fractures can result in a bone that grows noticeably shorter and more crooked than that of its opposing limb.

This is what happened to me.

Throughout this book, I've shared the stories of friends and clients. Now it's time to share my own. When I was a child, my hands were severely frostbitten, damaging the growth platelets in my hands. Even though I was only about twelve months old at the time, I still remember parts of the incident very lucidly. The rest I have learned from stories.

My father, who is a very attentive, loving man, took me outside to play during the winter. He wanted to keep an eye on me while he shoveled the snow from our driveway. Despite his best intent, I was alone in the icy-cold winter snow long enough to receive severe frostbite on both of my hands.

My parents immediately rushed me to our local hospital, where I was treated for my injuries, but by then, it was too late. My hands were already expanding like two balloons from the fluid buildup, and the damage had become so severe that the blood vessels on the inside of my fingers had begun to rupture and explode like a soda can someone had forgotten in the freezer. Unfortunately, the frostbite not only ruptured my blood vessels, but it also caused serious damage to the growth platelets in both of my hands.

The next thing I remember was screaming from the intense pain. The doctors were warming my fingers in a cool bath of water, and I was beginning to black out. I don't remember much from then on except that I needed several treatments to abrade the dead skin and fingernails from my damaged and broken hands.

As things calmed down over the next few years, there were concerns that my fingernails would never grow back. Fortunately, they did, but it became evident that I was going to have some very real problems from the accident.

I can't even remember how many doctor's appointments and physical therapy visits I had for my hands as a child, but due to the damaged growth platelets, my fingers were not able to grow to their full length. To make matters worse, my fingers and joints were now both growing crooked, creating an excessive amount of wear and tear to my finger joints and cartilage.

This caused me to develop severe degenerating arthritis in both of my hands. For many years, I struggled not only to fit in and feel wanted but to feel whole as a person. I began to search for alternative remedies to keep my hands both healthy and strong and to stop the destruction to my joints. But the arthritis kept on extirpating my joints until I was no longer able to use many of my fingers.

There were many days during this time when the pain and swelling were so bad that I couldn't even get out of bed. I was feverish, angry, and sick, and I would spend most of time in the bathroom vomiting from the pain. But I just kept thinking that if others could endure in the worst of circumstances, then I could too. I was tenacious in my efforts to overcome and to take care of myself and make a living no matter what. So, I taped my fingers into a fused position, downed a bunch a Tylenol, said a prayer, put a smile on my face, and went to work.

Despite my efforts, the pain and loss of function got worse, and I needed to explore my surgical options. A bone tumor had developed, which almost caused me to lose my left index finger. From the time I had that tumor removed until the time I was once again able to use my fingers more fully, I had endured eight surgeries in the period of about five years.

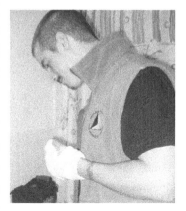

The surgeries corrected the pain in my most affected joints but at a cost: the surgeon had to remove my joints altogether and fuse my bones into a fixed position. There were concerns at the time that a conventional joint replacement could fail due to my high levels of physical activity, resulting in amputation of those fingers.

Regardless of whatever problems were going on with my hands at the time, I was constantly working to train my fitness clients, exercising whatever parts of my body I could despite my limitations, rigorously participating in my

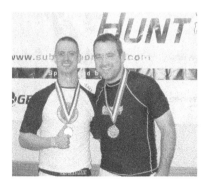

passion—martial arts—and trying to live a normal life. While the joint fusions did work, restoring an unbelievable quality of life, they also unfortunately reduced my ability to bend many of my fingers.

The extreme joint degeneration and the surgeries themselves also caused many additional unique problems. Every time I had a finger fixed, I had to re-learn how to use my hands. Each surgery cost a lot of money and left me feeling ill for months on end. And after every operation, I had to completely rebuild my body from the atrophy, struggling to perform the most basic daily tasks while my hands were healing. If I continued to have more surgeries to correct every one of my fingers, I would end up losing all of the mobility that I had left in my hands. This is always a pressing concern because I've had to leave some fairly affected joints alone to be able to use my hands.

I've been to some of the best specialists in the country to see what can be done about the rest of my fingers, but there is no way to fully correct the problem or judge how much time I will have left given the current state of the degeneration in my fingers. Plus, since I have surpassed all expectations, I tend to get the "ease up on your hands" speech. The doctors say I should take it easy if I want to live a longer life and get more use out of my hands as I get older.

But to me, it's about quality of life versus quantity. I have had to make some very stressful decisions about the course of my life, and this is a really heart-wrenching place to be in. There are only so many ways in which you can adapt your life and your activities before you have to make some extremely difficult decisions about what is most important to you.

Do you sacrifice everything that you enjoy, everything that you are, and everything that you will be for the sake of feeling some sense of security, knowing that even if you do, what you fear may come to pass anyway?

Or do you realize that, no matter what, if you can have just one more minute doing the things that are most important to you, and doing those things with the people that are the most important to you, it's all worth it in the end—even if you lose your physical independence?

I chose the latter, and I choose to do the things that I enjoy doing even if it makes my hands worse or speeds up my joint degeneration. I firmly believe in enjoying my life to the fullest. I would hate to live a long life and not enjoy any of it!

I've had to make this difficult choice every morning that I get out of bed, and every morning, I make the same decision. I make this choice because my greatest desire is that you would take something away from my experiences to make your life better!

If I can help you with even the smallest of my experiences, then every last second of pain, discomfort, and humiliation I've experienced has been worth it.

Perhaps you think to yourself, "I don't like the way that I look. I'm too fat. My butt is too big. My legs aren't skinny enough. If only I had a bigger chest or bigger muscles, I'd be happy." If any of these types of statements sound familiar, please stop putting yourself down. I have gone through all of this and more. I know what it's like to feel that your body sucks. I have had people say and do hurtful things or not want to be friends with me because of how I looked. Whatever you are going through, it's okay.

No matter what your body looks like, it's what makes you special and unique. I know that this won't magically make you feel better, but it's a start. You are not the only one who feels this way. We all have things about our bodies that we don't like, but the important thing to remember is that you are important and you can be loved no matter what you look like.

There is no need to feel down because you may look and feel different. If there are not a lot of people in your life right now praising you for who you are, then there's all the more of a reason for you to be singing your own praises.

When I was down and didn't feel good, I did the Stuart Smalley thing and gave myself pep talks in the mirror. I hated it at first, and I felt stupid because I thought that if other people knew, they would think that I was even weirder than I already felt. But in time, I really started to enjoy hearing those words of praise. It gave me confidence and strength. It made me feel bold, and it made me feel like I could want more for my life. But most importantly, it made me feel appreciated.

It is something small that you can do every day, and chances are that if you have identified with one of those negative statements about yourself, then you are already giving yourself pep talks. So, now all you have to do is to take it one small step at a time. It doesn't have to be all or nothing. Find something positive about yourself that you can believe in, and start from there. You can do it.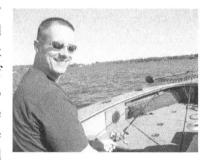

Remember to stay steady and stay strong. You are worth every second!

How to be Skinny Forever

Understanding Dietary Fat

Dietary Fat

Dietary fat is essential to a sound nutritional diet. It's vital to your health, and it's essential to your **Six-Week Body Challenge**. However, not all fatty acids are created equal, and for you to reap the full benefits of your body challenge, you will need to know the difference between good fats and bad. By knowing these differences, you will not only understand how your body processes fatty acids for use, but you will also understand my dietary recommendations for your fat consumption during **The Six-Week Body Challenge**. This will help you maintain your health and stay skinny forever!

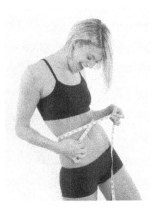

The Break Down

Fat is an essential nutrient for normal body function. It supplies your body with energy while also allowing you to absorb and utilize fat soluble vitamins A, D, E and K. Fat is important because it provides your body with the energy that it uses during low intensity, aerobic activities like sitting, walking, or jogging. If you've ever heard of the concept of exercising in a fat-burning zone, this is where it comes from. When you exercise at a lower intensity or in a fat-burning zone, fat is the primary source of energy for your body. The only downside is that the caloric expenditure is relatively low during these activities, making weight loss difficult with these types of exercises alone.

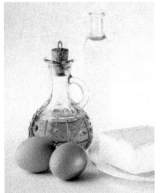

On a cellular level, fat is the foundation for forming healthy nerves and brain tissue. It also assists in maintaining proper cellular membrane structure and function. Fat maintains these structures by creating a border, keeping the things that belong inside your cells in and that which doesn't belong in your cells out. Fat is also essential for creating a proper hormone balance inside your body by keeping your hormonal organs healthy and strong.

However, the most important thing that fat does for **The Six-Week Body Challenge** is to contribute to satiety—the full feeling you have when you are done eating. This allows you to lose weight and avoid overeating. When examining the types of fats your body needs to be healthy and lose weight, not all fats are the same. There are three main types of fats: saturated, unsaturated and trans-fatty acids:

1. **Saturated Fats** are primarily found in animal sources, such as spare ribs, steak, and chicken with skin, and in dairy foods, like butter. With the exception of palm and coconut oil (which are also saturated fats), they are solid at room temperature (like lard or the fat on steak). Saturated fats are also the primary source of bad cholesterol. While consuming small amounts of saturated fats is good and healthy for the body, your intake of these types of fats should be kept to a minimum— no more than 30% of your total fat intake. If you are consuming 50 grams of fat for the day, then your intake of saturated fat should be 15 grams or less.

2. **Unsaturated fats** are found in plant and nuts sources and are liquid at room temperature. Olive oil is a good example of this. Unsaturated fats are structurally different than saturated fats, but they have the same caloric value: nine calories per gram. Examples of unsaturated fats are salad dressings, oils (except coconut and palm), margarine, mayonnaise, nuts, and avocados. Your daily intake of dietary fat should mainly consist of unsaturated fats.

3. **Trans Fats** come from adding hydrogen to vegetable oil through a process called hydrogenation. This creates hydrogenated and partially hydrogenated oils. Trans-fats are more solid than oil, making them less likely to spoil. By using trans-fatty acids, manufacturers are able to give their foods a longer shelf life. Trans-fatty acids also make foods feel less greasy.

   While trans-fatty acids are good for producing commercial goods and fried foods, trans-fatty acids raise your LDL (bad) cholesterol levels while simultaneously lowering your HDL (good) cholesterol levels.

Partially hydrogenated oils (trans-fats) may also increase inflammation in your body. Inflammation is the process by which your body responds to injury. While it is a necessary defense mechanism to guard against infection and help heal injury, excessive inflammation can lead to a body-wide response called sepsis, resulting in fever and organ failure. Inflammation also plays a key role in the formation of fatty blockages in your heart and blood vessels. You should try to avoid trans-fatty acids in your diet altogether.

Under-Consumption (Slow Metabolism)

Many people consider fat something bad to be avoided at all costs. They believe that any fat in food will become the fat that is stored in the body. This belief leads some extreme dieters to eating too little fat to maintain their body's vital processes and functions. While it is a good idea to cut down on saturated and trans-fatty acids, drastically reducing your intake of dietary fat in general is not a good idea.

Dietary fat supplies energy for your body, and consuming too little fat can cause you to lose energy throughout the day, making you feel sluggish and lethargic. Consuming too little dietary fat may actually slow down your metabolism, ironically causing your body to store more fat than it burns off for energy.

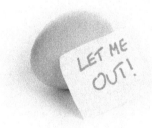

Fat is also extremely important for helping to regulate your blood sugar levels. When you eat, your blood sugar levels rise from your food consumption, especially when you eat carbohydrates. Fats and fatty acids keep your blood sugar levels from crashing and sending you into a hypoglycemic state. This is especially dangerous for diabetics, as this could cause them to experience a sugar crash at an unexpected time. Eating fat allows your metabolism to stabilize by increasing the time it takes for your food to break down while decreasing spikes and crashes in your blood sugar. Fat gives you consistent energy throughout the day.

When low or no-fat food substitutes are created by manufacturers, the fat in their products is replaced with other ingredients. Some of these ingredients are sugars and other processed carbohydrates. These ingredients have to be added because fat gives food its flavor, and without these sugars, the food would taste bland. However, these processed sugars can cause your body to store fat and increase your risk for health related illnesses like diabetes. So, how much fat should you consume on a daily basis?

How Much Fat Do You Need?

The average person needs to consume between 20 and 35% of his or her total daily calories from fat. The flexibility in this range helps you to determine how much fat you should be eating based on your level of physical activity. For the purposes of your body challenge, I have designed your menus to limit your fat intake to 25% of your total caloric needs.

● ● ● ● ● ● ● ● ● ● ●
Fat Activity Range:
20-25%: sedentary
to low activity
25-30%: moderately active
30-35%: highly active
● ● ● ● ● ● ● ● ● ● ●

Note: You should never consume less than 20% of your total calories from fat, or you can suffer from the negative side effects of under-consumption listed above.

For Men: Each week, your daily menu contains a total of 1,800 calories. Since 25% of those calories are coming from fat, you'll be consuming a total of 450 calories of fat every day. To convert that number into grams, divide your calories by nine instead of four. Unlike with protein and carbohydrates, for every gram of fat that you eat, you consume nine calories. Simply divide 450 by nine, and you need 50 grams of fat per day.

For Women: Each week, your daily menu contains a total of 1,400 calories, and because you are also consuming 25% of your total calories from fat, your total daily intake of fat should equal 350 calories. To convert this into grams, divide your intake of 350 calories by nine. This means that you need to consume roughly a total of 39 grams of fat each and every day to provide your body with the energy and nutrients it needs to be healthy and strong.

Your Fourth Menu

Menu Benefits (Increasing Your Omega-3 Intake)

Omega-3 fatty acids benefit the heart and those who are at risk for cardiovascular disease and stroke by acting as an anticoagulant and thinning the blood, similar to aspirin. Omega-3 fatty acids can also reduce inflammation, swelling and the formation of arterial plaque in the body.

This week's menu offers you a succulent herb-encrusted fish or chicken dish baked to a golden brown. It's also crammed full of fresh seafood and fish, free range chicken and eggs, and delicious whole grains to nourish your body with the rich Omega-3 foods you deserve!

Notes on This Week's Menu

Remember that it's okay to change the order of your meals as long as you make sure to stay with the same serving and portion sizes. It is also a good time to record your weight, take your measurements, and take follow-up pictures.

Your breakfast this week is intended to be two separate items. The eggs and cheese are intended to be one item, and the English muffin and peanut butter a separate item. I'm guessing that you figured this out, but I wanted to make sure you that you didn't feel as if you had to combine them. That might be a little gross!

Also, for your dinner, if you decide that you would like to do the couscous instead of the Jasmine Rice, the portion size should be the same for both the women's and men's menus. Simply use a quarter cup of dry couscous for the women and one third cup of dry couscous for the men. This will keep your calories roughly the same as the Jasmine rice.

No matter what you decide, it will taste great with your Herb and Macadamia Nut Encrusted Chicken or Fish dinner. Enjoy!

Special Entrée of the Week

Herb and Macadamia Nut Breading; this recipe perfectly complements your chicken or fish recipe by combining the great taste of macadamia nuts with the delicious taste of cracked bread crumbs and Italian herbs!

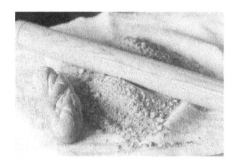 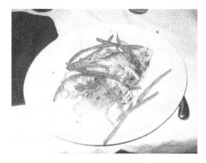

Macadamia Nut Herb Encrusted Chicken or Fish is a succulent macadamia nut herb encrusted chicken or fish dish baked to a golden brown and served with a side of green beans to ply your taste buds with delight!

Both recipes are available for only $0.99 each at:
CustomWorkoutVideos.com/catalog/index.php

get skinny!

Women's Menu: Week Four

Breakfast	Serving Size	Calories	Grams Protein Carbs, Fat	Comments
Liquid Egg Whites	1 serving (0.25 cup)	25 cal	5g protein, 1g carbs, 0g fat	based on Organic Valley liquid egg whites
Sharp Cheddar or Swiss Cheese Slice	0.5 slice (0.5oz)	55 cal	3.5g protein, 0g carbs, 4.5g fat	based on Trader Joes sharp cheddar cheese
English Muffin	0.5 muffin (1oz)	60 cal	2g protein, 12.5g carbs, 0.5g fat	based on Thomas Muffins
Creamy Peanut Butter	0.5 tbsp (0.3oz)	47 cal	2g protein, 1.75g carbs, 4g fat	based on Natural Creamy Jif

Snacks	Serving Size	Calories	Grams Protein Carbs, Fat	Comments
Peach Greek Yogurt	1 cup (6oz)	140 cal	14g protein, 20g carbs, 0g fat	based on no-fat Chobani brand yogurt
Strawberries	0.5 cups (3oz)	35 cal	0.5g protein, 6.5g carbs, 0.5g fat	based on an average organic brand
Granola Bar	0.5 package (1 bar)	80 cal	3g protein, 13g carbs, 2g fat	based on Nature Valley brand (apple crisp)

Lunch	Serving Size	Calories	Grams Protein Carbs, Fat	Comments
Low Carb Tortilla Shell	1 shell (2.2oz)	100 cal	8g protein, 17g carbs, 3.5g fat	based on La Tortilla Factory
Deli Meat Smoked Turkey or Roast Beef	1 serving (2oz)	60 cal	12g protein, 0g carbs, 3g fat	based on Applegate Farms deli meat

Sharp Cheddar or Swiss Cheese Slice	1 slice (1oz)	110 cal	7g protein, 0g carbs, 9g fat	based on Trader Joes sharp cheddar cheese
Butterhead Lettuce	2 slices (0.4oz)	<1cal	0g protein, <1g carbs, 0g fat	based on an average organic brand
Roma Tomatoes	4 slices (2.8oz)	14 cal	<1g protein, 3g carbs, 0g fat	based on an average organic brand
Yellow Mustard	1-2 tsp (0.2oz)	0 cal	0g protein, <1g carbs, 0g fat	based on French's classic yellow mustard

Snacks	Serving Size	Calories	Grams Protein Carbs, Fat	Comments
Granola Bar	0.5 package (1 bar)	80 cal	3g protein, 13g carbs, 2g fat	based on Nature Valley brand (apple crisp)
Banana	1 large (4.8oz)	136 cal	1.5g protein, 31g carbs, 0.5g fat	based on an average organic brand
Strawberries	0.5 cups (3oz)	35 cal	0.5g protein, 6.5g carbs, 0.5g fat	based on an average organic brand

Dinner	Serving Size	Calories	Grams Protein Carbs, Fat	Comments
*Herb and Macadamia Nut Encrusted Fish or Chicken	1 serving (5oz)	220 cal	27g protein, 12.5g carbs, 7g fat	Custom Workout Videos.com brand
Jasmine Rice or Couscous	0.25 cup (2oz)	160 cal	4g protein, 34g carbs, 2g fat	based on Lundberg's (uncooked Jasmine rice)

get skinny!

Men's Menu: Week Four

Breakfast	Serving Size	Calories	Grams Protein Carbs, Fat	Comments
Liquid Egg Whites	2 servings (0.5 cup)	50 cal	10g protein, 2g carbs, 0g fat	based on Organic Valley liquid egg whites
Sharp Cheddar or Swiss Cheese Slice	1 slice (1oz)	110 cal	7g protein, 0g carbs, 9g fat	based on Trader Joes sharp cheddar cheese
English Muffin	1 muffin (2oz)	120 cal	4g protein, 25g carbs, 1g fat	based on Thomas Muffins
Creamy Peanut Butter	1 tbsp (0.6oz)	95 cal	4g protein, 3.5g carbs, 8g fat	based on Natural Creamy Jif

Snacks	Serving Size	Calories	Grams Protein Carbs, Fat	Comments
Peach Greek Yogurt	1 cup (6oz)	140 cal	14g protein, 20g carbs, 0g fat	based on no-fat Chobani brand yogurt
Strawberries	1.5 cups (8.9oz)	105 cal	1.5g protein, 19.5g carbs, 0.5g fat	based on an average organic brand
Granola Bar	0.5 package (1 bar)	80 cal	3g protein, 13g carbs, 2g fat	based on Nature Valley brand (apple crisp)

Lunch	Serving Size	Calories	Grams Protein Carbs, Fat	Comments
Low Carb Tortilla Shell	1 shell (2.2oz)	100 cal	8g protein, 17g carbs, 3.5g fat	based on La Tortilla Factory
Deli Meat Smoked Turkey or Roast Beef	1.5 servings (3oz)	90 cal	18g protein, 0g carbs, 4.5g fat	based on Applegate Farms deli meat

Sharp Cheddar or Swiss Cheese Slice	1 slice (1oz)	110 cal	7g protein, 0g carbs, 9g fat	based on Trader Joes sharp cheddar cheese
Butterhead Lettuce	2 slices (0.4oz)	<1cal	0g protein, <1g carbs, 0g fat	based on an average organic brand
Roma Tomatoes	4 slices (2.8oz)	14 cal	<1g protein, 3g carbs, 0g fat	based on an average organic brand
Yellow Mustard	1-2 tsp (0.2oz)	0 cal	0g protein, <1g carbs, 0g fat	based on French's classic yellow mustard

Snacks	Serving Size	Calories	Grams Protein Carbs, Fat	Comments
Granola Bar	0.5 package (1 bar)	80 cal	3g protein, 13g carbs, 2g fat	based on Nature Valley brand (apple crisp)
Banana	1 large (4.8oz)	136 cal	1.5g protein, 31g carbs, 0.5g fat	based on an average organic brand
Strawberries	0.5 cups (3oz)	35 cal	0.5g protein, 6.5g carbs, 0.5g fat	based on an average organic brand

Dinner	Serving Size	Calories	Grams Protein Carbs, Fat	Comments
*Herb and Macadamia Nut Encrusted Fish or Chicken	1 serving (5oz)	220 cal	27g protein, 12.5g carbs, 7g fat	Custom Workout Videos.com brand
Jasmine Rice or Couscous	0.33 cup (2.4oz)	240 cal	6g protein, 51g carbs, 3g fat	based on Lundberg's (uncooked Jasmine rice)

Your Fourth Cardio Plan

Modifications and Benefits

The Benefits

Your fourth cardiovascular program is designed to accelerate the improvements in your circulatory system by helping your body build new blood vessels and by increasing your capillary density.

● ● ● ● ● ● ● ● ● ● ●

*Cardio Fun Fact: Capillaries are the smallest blood vessels in your body.

● ● ● ● ● ● ● ● ● ● ●

Capillaries are the tiny blood vessels which carry oxygen-rich blood to your body's tissues and cells, including muscle tissue. They are responsible for supplying the nutrients your body needs for maintenance and repair. Additionally, these tiny blood vessels absorb the carbon dioxide trapped in your cells and circulate the CO_2 out of your system via your veins and circulatory system.

Increasing capillary density is important for your **Six-Week Body Challenge**. Increased density will improve your exercise performance by increasing the amount of oxygen available to your muscle tissue. This will allow you to exercise more vigorously, burn more calories per workout, and increase your weight-loss potential. The increased capillary density from this cardio program paired with the increased stroke volume from last program will create greater cardiac output. This will help you to be able to take in more oxygen per breath and push out more blood per heartbeat. This means you can kick your program into high gear!

Your Fourth Cardio Program

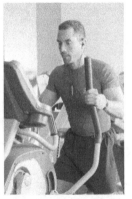

Your circuit training program this week involves challenging and developing your core strength and balance while making your arms and legs BURN! I want to make sure that your muscles are properly warmed and ready for the action. We'll be using the elliptical cross-trainer again to help us achieve these results.

Warm Up (7-10 min) Perform 7-10 minutes of light cardio on the elliptical before you start your workout routine, keeping your heart rate to be between 100-120 bpm. Working in this zone will properly warm up your body and oxygenate your muscle tissue to get you ready for your circuit training program. This heart rate training zone is about 50-55% of your maximum heart rate.

Cardio: End of Program (10-15 min) Do 10-15 minutes of cardio after your program. It's your time to really get your heart rate up and make major improvements to your heart and lungs, so keep your heart rate to be between 160-180 bpm.

This training zone is between 75-85% of your maximum heart rate, and working out at this intensity will make drastic improvements to your heart and lungs while burning a serious amount of calories. You will be breathing fairly heavily and won't to be able to speak in sentences. In fact, you'll probably struggle to speak altogether. Use these physiological cues to reinforce when you are training within the right zone.

You have been training hard the last three weeks, and you're ready for this intensity level. I want you to push yourself hard. You can do it. You are almost at the finish line, and I am proud of you for hanging in there and getting the job done!

Program Modifications

If you are still struggling with your level of cardiovascular conditioning and need modifications, you can alternate your heart rate on the elliptical between your training zone from this week (160-180bpm) and your training zone from last week (150-170bpm) until your time is finished. Alternate the intensities by going for one minute at the higher intensity and then for two minutes at the lower intensity until you're done. Make sure to slow down if you get dizzy, lightheaded or are unable to catch your breath.

Also, if you don't have access to an elliptical, here are some suggestions:

1. Go to your local community center or YMCA. They should have a cross-trainer you can use along with some space and exercise equipment you can use for your exercise routine afterward.

2. Go for a run or jog outside before your workout as long as it's warm out. If it is cold out, buy a jump rope and do your cardio at home. With a jump rope, it should be easy to get your heart rate up. No excuses!

Getting Stronger! Workout Four

What to Know

I am really excited about this program! It was fun to design, and I'm extremely proud of you for working so hard to get to this point!

This week's program is going to build on the huge improvements that you've been making to your core strength and flexibility, especially in your hips and glutes. When your hip muscles become tight and overused, your butt (gluteal) muscles will no longer work efficiently, even during basic daily activities. This will create a muscular imbalance, altering the way your body moves. Over time, it can cause a number of lower back, hip, and knee problems since your other muscles and joints have to work harder to compensate.

Here are some signs that may indicate that you're suffering from hip tightness, weak gluteal muscles, and pelvic instability:

1. A "bubble" butt, flat butt, or lack of definition in your butt muscles. Oh my!

2. An inability to keep your heels down while performing the squatting exercises in your body challenge.

3. Continual tightness and soreness in your lower back and hamstrings. This is very common if you're used to sitting or leaning forward for long periods of time, especially at your job.

4. Consistent pain in your knees (front or inside) and/or tenderness and pain in the front of your hips.

This week's exercises, specifically the Lateral Lunge, Modified Deadlift, and Overhead Squat, are designed to improve the strength and flexibility of your hip muscles, core musculature, and glutes. This will improve the rate at which your muscles fire. In personal training, this concept is called neuromuscular efficiency, which simply means that the muscles in your body are moving at the right time in relation to the muscles around them. Developing neuromuscular efficiency will not only benefit you in your body challenge, but it will also benefit you in your day-to-day activities as well as in sports like skiing, tennis, soccer, volleyball, and golf.

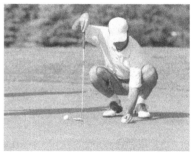

To help you understand how this week's program will help you increase your neuromuscular efficiency, let's take a look at the Modified Deadlift. When performing the Modified Deadlift, you start by engaging the core muscles in your stomach and back to elevate your chest. Next, you bend at your hips and then at your knees to sit back into a squat. (Your hip joint should always bend before your knees.) At the bottom of the deadlift, you focus on squeezing your glutes together, lifting through your heels, and driving your hips upward and forward. By learning the correct order and timing to contract your muscles during the Modified Deadlift, you can teach your body the neuromuscular efficiency needed to improve the strength and flexibility of your hips, core musculature, and glutes.

This is especially important if your glutes have become weak and lazy, because they may not automatically engage when you go to do simple activities like standing, squatting, walking, or running. While this may not sound serious, it puts excess pressure and stress on the surrounding muscles and joints, like your hips and knees. Then, what may start off as a minor amount of soreness can become something much more serious, such as a hamstring tear or a knee injury.

By using these exercises to teach your body how to move at its best, you will reduce your chances of developing an injury. You'll also give your body the strength and mobility it needs to do the activities you love!

Getting Stronger! Workout Four

Let's Get Started!!!

Getting Stronger! Workout Four

Protocol and Order:

- ◆ **(Warm Up)** Perform 7-10 minutes of cardio on the elliptical cross-trainer before you start your routine. Your heart rate should be between 100-120 bpm.

- ◆ **(Exercise)** Perform *two to three* circuits in order, keeping your heart rate between 140-160 bpm.

- ◆ **(Cardio)** Perform 10-15 minutes on the elliptical after your program with your heart rate between 160-180 bpm.

- ◆ **(Stretch)** Cool down using the stretches in this guide.

Duration: Week Four

Days per week: 2-3 (Leave 24 hours between sessions)

Exercise Reps: 10-12, 12-15, or 15-20, depending on the exercise

Load: Body weight or 45-55% 1 rep max

Circuits: 2-3

Rest interval: 15-30 seconds between exercises; 3-4 minutes between circuits

Equipment: Women: 9-12 lb body bar, two 5-8 lb dumbbells, two 10-12 lb dumbbells, two 12-15 lb dumbbells, and a 6 lb medicine ball

Men: 12-15 lb body bar, two 8-10 lb dumbbells, two 10-12 lb dumbbells, two 15-20 lb dumbbells, and an 8 lb medicine ball

Note: The last few reps on each exercise should be taxing. When you can comfortably perform the number of repetitions suggested, increase your weight.

Lateral Lunge # 1

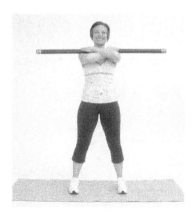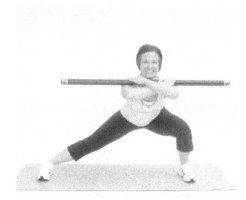

a. **(Part 1)** Stand upright with your feet slightly wider than shoulder-width apart. Grab the body bar first with your left hand and then with your right so that your right arm is over your left. While holding onto the bar, lift your chest up and raise your elbows until they're parallel to the floor, letting the bar rest on top of your shoulders. (The bar should remain horizontal throughout the exercise.)

b. **(Part 2)** Lunge laterally to one side while moving your hips in the same direction, straightening out your supporting leg as you do. Land by planting onto your lunging foot, and then lean back onto your heel.

c. Make sure to lunge into a wide stance. This will allow you adequate room to move your hips backward while keeping your lunging knee behind your toes to prevent knee strain.

d. **(Part 3)** Keep your supporting leg extended as you lower your body by bending at your knees while sticking your butt out. Continue to lower your body until the knee and hip of your lunging leg are parallel to one another. Keep your chest up and at a 45° angle to your hips when squatting. This is to avoid any rounding in the back, which can cause lower back pain.

e. **(Part 4)** Once you've attained a full range of motion, return to the starting position by driving your hips upward and forward until your hips are aligned in a with your spine.

f. Your back should remain flat throughout the movement with your chest up. Return and repeat all repetitions to one side before switching.

Special Instructions:

Before you begin performing this exercise dynamically by lunging side-to-side, practice squatting in the ending position, with one leg straight. Do this eight to ten times on each side to get familiar with the movement before you begin.

Perform: 10-12 repetitions (each side) – hands in front squat position
Women: 9-12 lb body bar
Men: 12-15 lb body bar

Modified (Sumo Squat) Deadlift # 2

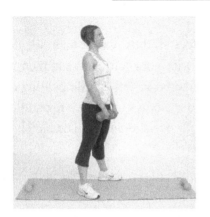 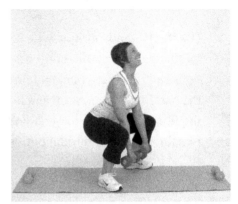

a. **(Part 1)** Stand with your feet slightly wider than your shoulder-width apart, and turn your toes out until your knees are in line with your hips. Squat down by sticking your butt out while elevating your chest to avoid rounding your back.

b. As you bend down, hold your dumbbells down between your legs, letting your arms move along the inside of your legs. Continue to squat until the points of your elbows touch the inside of your thighs.

c. **(Part 2)** Keeping your chest elevated, exhale and gently thrust your hips forward while contracting your hamstrings and glutes until your body is upright. Keep your back flat as you lift off the floor and extend through your heels. Repeat.

Perform: 10-12 repetitions
Women: 12-15 lb dumbbells (each hand)
Men: 15-20 lb dumbbells (each hand)

Overhead Squat # 3

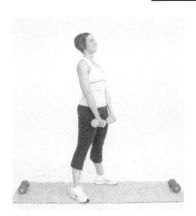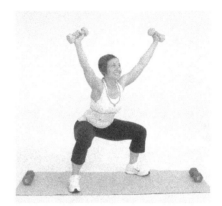

a. **(Part 1)** Stand with your feet slightly wider than shoulder-width apart and turn your toes out so your hips and knees are in a straight line. Grab two dumbbells and, with a slight bend in your elbows, drop your arms down by your knees with your palms facing your legs.

b. **(Part 2)** Lower your body by bending at your knees while sticking your butt out. Lower your body until your hips and knees are parallel. Keep your chest up and at a 45° angle to your hips when squatting.

c. While squatting, raise both dumbbells up and back until you can squeeze your shoulder blades together. Use your legs, your back and the rest of your core muscles to stabilize your body position.

d. **(Part 3)** While you're standing up, drive your hips forward until you can squeeze your butt cheeks together and until your hips are aligned with your spine. Drop the dumbbells. Repeat.

Perform: 12-15 repetitions
Women: 5-8 lb dumbbells (each hand)
Men: 8-10 lb dumbbells (each hand)

Medicine Ball Slam # 4

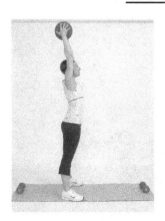 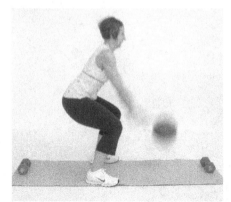

a. Stand with your feet slightly wider than shoulder-width apart and turn your toes out until your knees and hips are in a straight line.

b. Grab a medicine ball between your hands, pull it back behind your head, and hold it at arm's length overhead.

c. Forcefully throw the ball down on the ground as hard as possible while squatting down at the same time. (Keep your arms straight while slamming the ball.)

d. Catch the ball as it bounces up from the ground. Stand up, return to starting position, and repeat.

Special Instructions:

This is a timed exercise. Complete all of your reps in 20-25 seconds.

Perform: 15-20 repetitions
Women: 6 lb medicine ball
Men: 8 lb medicine ball

Upright Row # 5

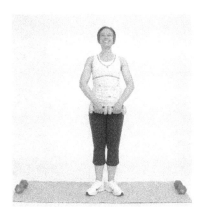 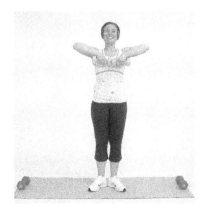

a. Stand with your back upright and feet together in a V-shape with legs and glutes contracted.

b. Extend your arms downward with wrists and elbows in a straight line and palms facing toward your body.

c. Raise the weights by bending your elbows upward. Move them along your body until your elbows are at a 90° angle and parallel with the floor.

d. Hold and return the dumbbells down your body the same way you brought them up. Repeat.

Special Instructions:

Keep your elbows elevated and above your wrists while you are lifting the weights.

Perform: 12-15 repetitions
Women: 5-8 lb dumbbells (each hand)
Men: 10-12 lb dumbbells (each hand)

Bicep Curl to Press # 6

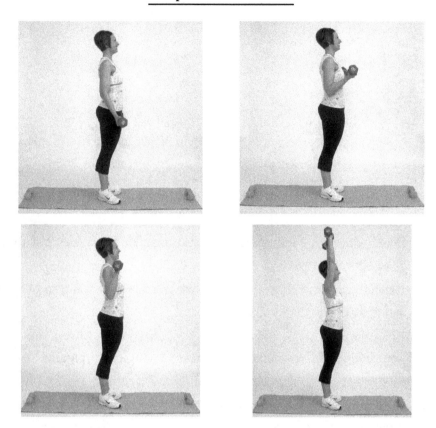

a. **(Part 1)** Hold a dumbbell in each hand with a soft grip, weights at your sides and palms facing upward.

b. Stand with your back upright and feet together in a V-shape with legs and glutes contracted. Keep your back upright, shoulders relaxed and your elbows in.

c. Slowly raise the weights by bending your elbows inward until your knuckles are 3-4 inches away from your shoulders. Turn your palms facing outward.

d. **(Part 2)** Look up and inhale while pressing to keep your spine straight. Stop when your arms are extended straight overhead. Keep your wrists, shoulders and elbows in a straight line.

e. Exhale and slowly lower the weights back to the starting position in the same way you pressed up.

Perform: 10-12 repetitions
Women: 10-12 lb dumbbells (each hand)
Men: 15-20 lb dumbbells (each hand)

Your Fourth Stretching Routine

Now that you're done with your workout, let's cool down!

What to Know

Your fourth exercise program is designed to build up the strength of your gluteal muscles and core strength while improving the rate at which your muscles fire.

To compliment these exercises, the stretches in your fourth routine will reduce any tightness that you may experience in your gluteal and core muscles after you're done working out. These stretches will also help to loosen the muscles in your shoulders and get your upper body ready for the exercises in your fifth workout program.

Sitting Trap Stretch

- Sit on a balance ball and put your right arm between your legs with your upper arm pressed against your thigh.

- Twist your torso, lift your left arm up in the air until your shoulders are in line with one another, and look up.

Stretching Benefits:

The muscles of your mid-back and trapezius attach to your neck. When these muscles get tight, they can cause stiffness, headaches, and neck pain.

Perform: 2 sets of 1 repetition
Sides: Both
Hold stretch for 30 seconds.

Standing Side Stretch

- Stand with your legs wide apart with your right leg out in front.

- Point your right toes straight forward and your left toes out until your feet make a T-shape.

- Twist and place your right elbow on your thigh, straighten your left arm up, and stretch toward the opposite wall.

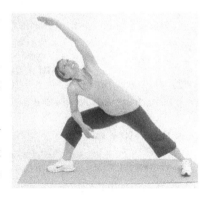

Stretching Benefits:

Tight latissimus dorsi muscles will cause your shoulder blades to rotate forward, leading to pain and dysfunction of the shoulder joint.

Perform: 2 sets of 1 repetition
Sides: Both
Hold stretch for 30 seconds.

Side Lying Quad Stretch

- Lie on one side, grab your ankle or foot, and bend your knee backward.

- Straighten your hip by pulling your ankle or foot backward, keeping your knee bent. Don't let your knee extend too far upward beyond your hip.

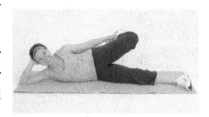

Stretching Benefits:

Tight quadriceps muscles can cause stiffness and lower back pain by pulling your pelvis forward out of its natural alignment.

Perform: 2 sets of 1 repetition
Sides: Both
Hold stretch for 30 seconds.

Hamstring Stretch

- Keep your back upright.

- Straighten one leg while tucking the other in.

- Lean forward with your back upright until you are comfortably stretching the backside of your leg.

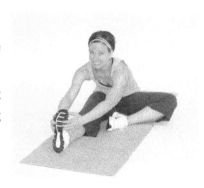

Stretching Benefits:

Tight hamstring muscles can cause your lower legs to twist outward in the direction of your toes, putting pressure on your joints and causing pain.

Perform: 2 sets of 1 repetition
Sides: Both
Hold stretch for 30 Seconds.

Lying Piriformis Stretch

- Lie down on your back and cross your right leg over your left.

- Reach through your legs to grab your left leg and pull it towards your chest.

- Use your right elbow to push on your right knee until you feel the stretch in your gluteal muscle on the right side.

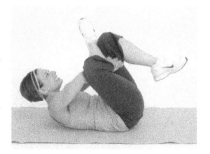

Stretching Benefits:

Tight piriformis muscles can put pressure on your sciatic nerves, causing pain.

Perform: 2 sets of 1 repetition
Sides: Both
Hold stretch for 30 seconds.

Ball-Lying Chest Stretch

- Lie with your back on a balance ball.
- Roll down until your head and neck are fully supported.
- Relax your hips and let your arms fall out to your sides.

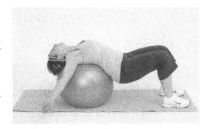

Stretching Benefits:

Tight chest muscles can cause Upper Cross Syndrome or rounded shoulders, which can lead to bursitis, a shoulder impingement or a rotator cuff injury.

Perform: 2 sets of 1 repetition
Hold stretch for 30 seconds.

Chapter 5

mirror, mirror on the wall

Her Emotional Path of Self-Discovery

My name is Kristi, and I was extremely overweight and unhappy while I was growing up. I always felt that I stood out amongst my slimmer friends.

Although I was never a very petite girl, I tried to be athletic to stay in shape, especially because I had a pear-shaped body, which kind of made me feel self-conscious about my looks. I felt like I stood out so much from my other skinny friends and that people would judge me.

I was also really pretty growing up, but I never felt confident about myself because my legs and body didn't portray the ideal standards of beauty that I saw around me, especially in magazines and on television. I would buy into these unrealistic standards of beauty because of my lack of confidence. I wasn't sure if other people saw me as a fun and pretty girl or if I was simply the big girl with the pretty face.

I struggled so much that when I went from grade school to middle school at age 11, I gained a lot of weight. I was convinced that the only way I could feel better about myself was to be skinny like the more popular girls around me. I had to lose weight, so I started playing three sports at a time. I played softball and soccer in the summers, and I played hockey in the winter. I found that I also loved playing volleyball, but I quit playing when I got to high school because the uniform included tight spandex shorts. There was no way I was ever going to let anyone see me in tight shorts, especially with my big legs.

I tried dieting and skipping meals to lose weight in addition to sports, but no matter how hard I tried, these things only made me feel worse about myself for being fake. I wasn't addressing the real issue that was going on: how I felt about *me*. This only ended up making me feel more down on myself. I felt cursed to be like this when others didn't seem to even have to try. I felt like all I had to do was *look* at food and gain weight while other girls could do whatever they wanted without gaining a single pound. It all felt really unfair.

It was an ache lodged deep inside of me at both a physical and an emotional level. The more depressed I felt, the more I would eat. It was a vicious cycle of pain and regret. My only sense of sanity in this was telling myself that it wasn't that bad, and that come tomorrow or Monday, I could start over. Then, Monday would come and I would be good for a few days until something would set me off, and I would eat a bunch of junk. Figuring that my whole week was now ruined, I would give up and blow my diet big, simply to start the cycle all over again the next week.

This continued all the way through high school, only it was worse because there were fewer sports available for me to play while I was there. This added fuel to the fire.

When I was 20 years old, I bought my first house and ended up in a dead-end relationship. I was so excited about getting married and having a family, but my fiancé was not excited about anything in his life. He constantly sat around the house while I was at work, and he expected me to take care of him like some sort of man-child. He would play on the computer all day and go out with his friends at night, but he did nothing to support himself or our relationship. It drained me physically and emotionally so much that I resorted to eating as a way of dealing with what was going on.

Finally, I was able to gather the strength to tell him that things weren't going to work out for us. I needed someone who would love and support me, not just look to me as his source of income. But because of the weight that I had gained from this experience, I developed another nightmare in my life. My legs and butt were becoming so big that shopping for clothes, especially jeans, became a really miserable experience.

I was afraid to try anything on because, deep down, I knew that it meant that I had to face what was going on. But after dealing with the hurt of coming out of that bad relationship and living with the pain of how big I was becoming, I simply wasn't ready to face my problems.

I convinced myself that the styles and brands that I was trying on were to blame instead of my weight, but it became more and more difficult to find anything that would fit me. The sizes I needed just kept getting bigger and bigger. Then, when I would finally summon the courage to try on something new, I always wanted to get a smaller size than I needed. I felt horrible in the dressing room because I couldn't fit into anything. It made the whole situation seem like such a lost cause.

After trying on one outfit after another for hours on end, I would leave the mall empty-handed, feeling really frustrated and defeated.

I had always felt like there was something wrong with me, like I was cursed. Every time I had experiences like this, it just reaffirmed that I was somehow different. I couldn't understand why I felt so alone or why this was happening to me. It was as if I was being punished for something I didn't deserve. I would completely break down and cry after I had gotten home because the reality of my weight problem was undeniable.

Things went on like this for what felt like an eternity. Then, just like that, something wonderful happened to me. A cousin of mine introduced me to a really cute guy at her work.

This is how I met my best friend and significant other. We got along so well that we started dating almost right away. Before I even knew what was going on, I started to feel good about myself again. But when it came to losing weight, things were still tough for me.

My boyfriend travels a lot for his job, and he loves to eat out. Even when he's at home, he wants to eat junk food. Although I wanted to change, it was really tempting to eat junk food with him.

Things at work were also prompting me to make a change. As a dental hygienist, I spend the better part of my day hunched over patients. My work had really started to take a toll on my back and shoulders, which made me want to get in shape to strengthen my body. I was also becoming aware of how many of my family members were overweight and had heart problems and diabetes. My grandpa had a heart attack when he was only 57 years old, so it was always in the back of my mind that I could be dealing with a lifelong problem of high blood pressure, heart disease, and diabetes if I didn't make a change.

This is when I met Scott. I had joined a local gym at my mom's recommendation. She'd recently begun her own weight-loss journey with Scott and mentioned how much she liked him. She told me to come along during one of her sessions and have him take a look at my back and shoulders to see if he could help while also helping me lose some weight.

When we first started working out, I didn't realize just how out of shape I was. I thought I was fine because I would occasionally do some stretching along with a few pushups and sit ups around the house. But I was huffing and puffing just trying to get through my warm-up! I wasn't even able to get through all of the core exercises Scott wanted me to do at first. Fortunately, my back began to feel better after just a few sessions, which made me want to continue despite my poor performance.

I expected Scott to yell at me and call me names like a drill sergeant, but he never berated me for being out of shape. Instead, he simply modified the exercises for me so I could still complete them successfully and feel good about myself. Of course, that doesn't mean he ever made it easy for me. Whenever I was having a hard time and didn't feel like I could do anymore, Scott would look at me with this evil grin on his face and encourage me to push myself.

I always knew it was going to be a tough workout when he would say, "We are going to have a really fun session today," especially when he had that mischievous grin on his face. But no matter what, Scott never gave up on me. He pushed me to reach my inner potential. This made me feel confident enough to make mistakes and learn from them. By not letting me settle, Scott forced me to remember why I had wanted to get in shape in the first place and taught me to be consistent.

Before I worked with Scott, I had been selectively picking my way through dieting and exercise in a manner that was so inconsistent. I was only eating healthy a few times a week until something came up that completely derailed me, and I was really only doing a few pushups and sit ups here and there, which hardly counts as exercise. No wonder I wasn't seeing results!

I knew I had to push myself if I was ever going to be successful because eating healthy and exercising isn't always easy. I still love junk foods and indulgences, but I don't eat them all the time like I did before.

Life gets in the way, and there are always going to be temptations and struggles to overcome. And even though I have put a little weight back on since I have finished training with Scott, he has helped me tremendously. I have learned a much better way of dealing with the frustrations in my life, I eat so much better and cleaner than ever before, and I am really consistent about my exercise. I have even found a workout partner to go with me to the gym.

Having a workout partner who is extremely consistent about showing up (and not just consistent about finding reasons to cancel) has really helped motivate me. I am not just working out for myself anymore! We meet each other at the gym almost every morning before work to go running, and we line up our schedules so we can take two exercise classes a week outside of our morning routine.

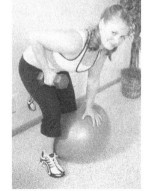

I have not only lost the perfect amount of weight for me, but, more importantly, I have learned to be completely comfortable with my own body and who I am. It turns out that even skinny girls have things about their bodies that they like to criticize!

I am happier than ever before, and I can honestly say that no matter how bad you may feel right now, please don't give up on yourself. You can be happy too!

Salt's a Bloat

Understanding Sodium and Chloride

Table Salt

Salt is not only essential to human life but also to good health. It is composed of two electrically composed particles, sodium and chloride. These particles, also called electrolytes, work alongside potassium, water and other electrolytes to maintain the function of your nerves, muscles, and cells. Most importantly for your **Six-Week Body Challenge**, these electrolytes work to keep you well-hydrated and feeling strong.

The Break Down

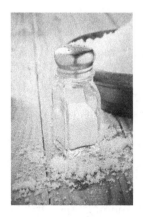

Your muscle tissue requires electricity and electrical currents to contract, and your cells create these contractions by altering your concentrations of ions or "electrolytes" in your body – specifically sodium and potassium. It's important to have a sufficient level of sodium and potassium in your system when exercising, or you will fatigue easily and experience intense muscle cramping. Maintaining your electrolyte levels becomes even more important when you're exercising in warm or hot weather. If you don't, you'll start to feel light-headed, nauseous or disoriented. Low levels of sodium can also interfere with your body's ability to stay cool when exercising, leading to heat stroke, or it can interfere with the nerve impulses in your brain, potentially causing a seizure.

Sore muscles and leg cramps during exercise are also a sign that your electrolytes levels are low and your intensity level is high. Severe muscle cramps can cause damage to your muscle tissue by causing your muscle fibers to tear under the strength of their own contractions. Salt helps to maintain your need to drink water and your levels of hydration while working with the glucose in your body to enhance the absorption rate of the water in your intestines. This increases your rate of hydration.

On the other hand, consuming too much sodium can negatively impact your body as well.

Over-Consumption (High Blood Pressure and a Bloated Belly)

Your kidneys are responsible for regulating the amount of sodium stored within your body. As your sodium levels start to rise, your kidneys excrete the excess out through your urine. If you start consuming more sodium than your kidneys can excrete, then the sodium levels in your blood stream will increase, which will force your body to compensate by retaining water to help your kidneys flush it out. This whole process will leave you feeling bloated and gross and will cause your stomach to bulge out because of the excess water retention. Yuck!

In addition to bloating, water retention also increases your blood pressure. This forces your heart to work much harder than normal to pump out blood, which puts extra pressure against your arterial walls. It's important to note that some people are more sensitive to sodium than others, so it takes 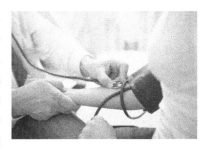 them much less sodium to experience these side-effects. In extreme cases, excess sodium levels can lead to congestive heart failure, kidney disease, and stroke.

How Much Salt Do You Need?

Healthy adults should not consume more than 2,300 milligrams (mg) per day. (This amount is equal to one teaspoon of table salt.) Individuals who suffer from heart and kidney disease, high blood pressure, or diabetes should not consume more than 1,500mg of sodium per day.

The U.S. Department of Agriculture estimates that the average American consumes more than 4,000 milligrams (mg) of sodium every day, which is far more than the recommended daily allowance for a healthy adult. They also believe that most people are not getting their salt from the salt shaker. So, where is it coming from?

Most of the extra salt that we consume each day comes from eating out at restaurants or from eating pre-packaged, processed and store-bought foods. The next time you go out for dinner, ask to see if they have any low salt, no-salt substitutions, and remember to read the nutrition labels on foods you like to purchase at the grocery store. You might just be surprised at how much sodium these products contain. Also, try adding in more fresh, unprocessed foods like fruits and vegetables. They are naturally low in sodium and high in cancer-fighting antioxidants.

Your Fifth Menu

Menu Benefits (Low Sodium Diet)

A diet that is low in sodium and high in fiber can reduce your risk of heart disease and stroke and can be part of a heart healthy plan to lower blood pressure. Also, for those who suffer from kidney disease, a diet that is low sodium is critical to the prevention of fluid retention and swelling within your body.

As a part of our heart healthy plan, this week's menu offers a deliciously satisfying dish of orange spices and farm-fresh meat. It's also brimming with low-sodium foods like fresh fruits and vegetables, rich whole grains, and heart healthy eggs to give your body the loving it needs!

Notes on This Week's Menu

The same rules apply for changing the order of your meals this week. Also, remember to record your weight, take your measurements, and take follow-up pictures.

This week, you can substitute rice noodles for Jasmine rice. Just make sure that your portion size comes out to three-quarters cup of cooked noodles for women and one cup of cooked noodles for men. This will keep your calories roughly the same as the Jasmine rice.

Special Entrée of the Week

Herbs, Orange Spice and Everything Nice offers you a deliciously satisfying dish that will indulge your cravings for exotic cuisine with its tempting orange spices and delectable chunks of farm fresh meats!

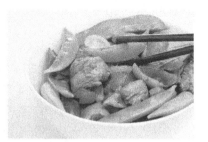

This recipe is available for only $0.99 at:
CustomWorkoutVideos.com/catalog/index.php

Note: This dish has some hot peppers to create additional flavor, but if you don't like spicy dishes, you can remove them. This dish tastes just as good to cook it without the hot spices.

Women's Menu: Week Five

Breakfast	Serving Size	Calories	Grams Protein Carbs, Fat	Comments
English Muffin	0.5 muffin (1oz)	60 cal	2g protein, 12.5g carbs, 0.5g fat	based on Thomas Muffins
Creamy Peanut Butter	0.5 tbsp (0.6oz)	47 cal	2g protein, 1.75g carbs, 4g fat	based on Natural Creamy Jif
Chocolate Almond Milk	1 cup (8oz)	105 cal	1.5g protein, 18g carbs, 3g fat	based on Blue Diamond brand milk

Snacks	Serving Size	Calories	Grams Protein Carbs, Fat	Comments
Raspberry Greek Yogurt	1 cup (6oz)	140 cal	14g protein, 20g carbs, 0g fat	based on no-fat Chobani brand yogurt
Blueberries	0.5 cup (2.5oz)	41 cal	0.5g protein, 11g carbs, 0g fat	based on an average organic brand
Granola Bar	0.5 package (1 bar)	80 cal	3g protein, 13g carbs, 2g fat	based on Nature Valley brand (apple crisp)

Lunch	Serving Size	Calories	Grams Protein Carbs, Fat	Comments
Rosemary Olive Oil Bread	2 slices (2.8oz)	200 cal	8g protein, 40g carbs, 2g fat	based on Rudi's Organic (can be changed for wheat bread, any brand)
Deli Meat Smoked Turkey or Roast Beef	1 serving (2oz)	60 cal	12g protein, 0g carbs, 3g fat	based on Applegate Farms deli meat

Sharp Cheddar or Swiss Cheese Slice	1 slice (1oz)	110 cal	7g protein, 0g carbs, 9g fat	based on Trader Joes sharp cheddar cheese
Butterhead Lettuce	2 slices (0.4oz)	<1cal	0g protein, <1g carbs, 0g fat	based on an average organic brand
Roma Tomatoes	4 slices (2.8oz)	14 cal	<1g protein, 3g carbs, 0g fat	based on an average organic brand
Yellow Mustard	1-2 tsp (0.2oz)	0 cal	0g protein, <1g carbs, 0g fat	based on French's classic yellow mustard

Snacks	Serving Size	Calories	Grams Protein Carbs, Fat	Comments
Chocolate Fudge Brownie	1 bar	90 cal	1g protein, 18g carbs, 3g fat	based on Fiber One Brand

Dinner	Serving Size	Calories	Grams Protein Carbs, Fat	Comments
*Herbs, Orange Spice and Everything Nice	1 serving (5oz)	284 cal	40g protein, 15g carbs, 8g fat	Custom Workout Videos.com brand
Jasmine Rice or Rice Noodles	0.25 cup (2oz)	160 cal	4g protein, 34g carbs, 2g fat	based on Lundberg's (uncooked Jasmine rice)

Men's Menu: Week Five

Breakfast	Serving Size	Calories	Grams Protein Carbs, Fat	Comments
English Muffin	1 muffin (2oz)	120 cal	4g protein, 25g carbs, 1g fat	based on Thomas Muffins
Creamy Peanut Butter	1.5 tbsp (0.6oz)	143 cal	6g protein, 5.25g carbs, 12g fat	based on Natural Creamy Jif
Chocolate Almond Milk	1.5 cups (12oz)	140 cal	2g protein, 24g carbs, 4g fat	based on Blue Diamond brand milk

Snacks	Serving Size	Calories	Grams Protein Carbs, Fat	Comments
Raspberry Greek Yogurt	1 cup (6oz)	140 cal	14g protein, 20g carbs, 0g fat	based on no-fat Chobani brand yogurt
Blueberries	0.5 cup (2.5oz)	41 cal	0.5g protein, 11g carbs, 0g fat	based on an average organic brand
Granola Bar	0.5 package (1 bar)	80 cal	3g protein, 13g carbs, 2g fat	based on Nature Valley brand (apple crisp)

Lunch	Serving Size	Calories	Grams Protein Carbs, Fat	Comments
Rosemary Olive Oil Bread	2 slices (2.8oz)	200 cal	8g protein, 40g carbs, 2g fat	based on Rudi's Organic Bakery (can be changed for any wheat bread)
Deli Meat Smoked Turkey or Roast Beef	1.5 servings (3oz)	90 cal	18g protein, 0g carbs, 4.5g fat	based on Applegate Farms deli meat

Sharp Cheddar or Swiss Cheese Slice	1 slice (1oz)	110 cal	7g protein, 0g carbs, 9g fat	based on Trader Joes sharp cheddar cheese
Butterhead Lettuce	2 slices (0.4oz)	<1cal	0g protein, <1g carbs, 0g fat	based on an average organic brand
Roma Tomatoes	4 slices (2.8oz)	14 cal	<1g protein, 3g carbs, 0g fat	based on an average organic brand
Yellow Mustard	1-2 tsp (0.2oz)	0 cal	0g protein, <1g carbs, 0g fat	based on French's classic yellow mustard

Snacks	Serving Size	Calories	Grams Protein Carbs, Fat	Comments
Chocolate Fudge Brownie	1 bar	90 cal	1g protein, 18g carbs, 3g fat	based on Fiber One Brand
Orange or Apple	1 small (3.4oz)	50 cal	1g protein, 11.5g carbs, 0g fat	based on an average organic brand

Dinner	Serving Size	Calories	Grams Protein Carbs, Fat	Comments
*Herbs, Orange Spice and Everything Nice	1 serving (5oz)	284 cal	40g protein, 15g carbs, 8g fat	Custom Workout Videos.com brand
Jasmine Rice or Rice Noodles	0.33 cup (2.4oz)	240 cal	6g protein, 51g carbs, 3g fat	based on Lundberg's (uncooked Jasmine rice)

Your Fifth Cardio Plan

Modifications and Benefits

Benefits

Your fifth cardiovascular program is designed to improve your joint health. As you get older, your joints can become swollen and painful. This may cause you to want to limit your levels of physical activity. However, avoiding physical activity because of joint pain will cause significant muscle loss and lead to excessive weight gain.

This program is extremely effective for reducing joint pain and improving function. Using the upright bike will take the weight and pressure off of your joints, and the repetitive motion will help to restore your mobility by increasing the temperature of your joint fluid. Joint fluid or synovial fluid is similar to a thick paste or gel. When it is warmed up through physical activity, it becomes thinner and acts as a better lubricant, reducing the amount of wear and tear in your joints. This is the reason why people who suffer from arthritis experience more joint pain than normal on a cool, frigid day. (The fluid within their joints becomes thicker and has a tougher time acting as a lubricant.) Using the upright bike also helps to build up the muscle tissue in your thighs around your knees, creating more support for your joints.

Improving your joint health will allow you to become more physically active, burn more calories, and lose weight. This is especially helpful as losing weight will also help take the pressure off of your joints, leading to more freedom and mobility!

Your Fifth Cardio Program

Your circuit training program this week involves increasing your arm and shoulder strength while improving your flexibility through dynamic motion. Accomplishing this program will require the intensive use of your core to stabilize your body and lower back. To get your lower body and core ready for your program, we will be using the upright bike!

Warm Up (7-10 min) Warm up by performing 7-10 minutes of cardio on the upright bike before you engage in your workout routine. I want your heart rate to be between 100-120 bpm. This zone will get your lower body and core properly oxygenated and ready for your circuit training routine.

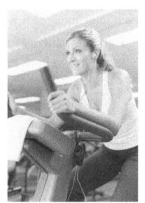

Cardio: End of Program (10-15 min) Do 10-15 minutes of cardio after your program. We have two more weeks (counting this week) to help you lose weight, so let's work hard this week and get your heart rate up between 140-160 bpm. This is between 60-70% of your maximum heart rate. This training zone will improve your joint function and health while still allowing for improvements in your cardiovascular system.

During your cardio program, you will still be able to speak, but in only small sentences. Your rate of breathing is going to become much heavier than during your warm-up, but you won't be breathing as heavily and as fast as you did during your cardio program last week. It might even feel like you are not going as hard, and you may want to speed up, but it's okay to have a slower week, especially for your joint's sake. Use these physiological cues to help reinforce when you are training at the right intensity. Remember, you have only two weeks to go. Stay Focused. You can do it!

Program Modifications

You should be noticing some drastic improvements in your level of cardiovascular conditioning, and you may not need modifications, especially at this intensity. So, for this week, I am just going to list some modifications in the event that you don't have access to an upright bike. However, if you do get dizzy, lightheaded or are unable to catch your breath, please slow down long enough for the feeling to pass and then resume at your normal training intensity for this week.

If you don't have access to an upright bike, here are some suggestions:

1. Bring your heart rate monitor along and go for a bike ride outside.

2. Go for a light jog outside, weather permitting, but keep your intensity down to the recommended heart rate training zone. This will help with

your joints, especially as all-out running on hard, uneven surfaces may cause some discomfort.

3. If you have good weather and access to a pool, go swimming. You won't be able to wear your heart rate monitor, so make sure to use your physiological cues for this activity, and make sure the pool is heated to between 83 and 88° Fahrenheit. At this temperature, the water should feel soothing but not hot. Anything colder than this temperature will make it difficult to get your joints warmed up.

4. Go to your local community center or YMCA. They should have an upright bike you can use along with some space and exercise equipment you can use for your exercise routine afterward.

Almost There! Workout Five

What to Know

This week's program will be invaluable to developing the strength and mobility in your upper back and shoulders. Fully developing this musculature will protect your shoulder joints from injury.

While you probably don't think much about your upper body on a daily basis, your shoulders are unique and prone to injury because of their structure. In fact, your body's movements are actually based on these individual structures. For example, your hips are required to support the weight of your entire upper body while providing locomotion to your lower body, so they must have an enclosed structure (ball and socket joint) with limited mobility to prevent dislocation.

However, because your shoulder joints have to accommodate for a much wider range of motion than your hips, they are comprised of a less enclosed version of a ball and socket joint, which is mainly held together by muscle and tendon. It is this unique joint structure that gives your upper body its freedom of movement, especially when compared to the mobility of your lower body and hips. But this unique structure also causes your shoulders to be significantly less stable than your hips, making your shoulders far more prone to injury and dislocation.

The main thing that you can do to prevent your shoulders from being injured or dislocated is to build up the strength and mobility of your upper back and shoulders. This will keep you from having weak postural muscles in your back, which is one of the main reasons why your shoulders round forward.

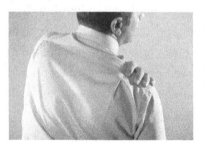

The other main reason is frequent, repetitive stress like reaching out and overhead when doing activities such as yard work, driving, or working on the computer without elbow support.

Repetitive stress from being hunched forward will put pressure on your shoulders and spine, especially as the big muscles in your chest (pectoralis muscles) and back (latissimus dorsi) become tight and shortened. Left unchecked, this will lead to several problems in your upper back, as the small muscles between your shoulder blades are not designed to support the weight of your upper body. This will force these muscles to stretch out and grow weak, causing pain and increasing your chances of developing an injury. This can also cause several problems of the spine like osteoarthritis or a herniated disc from the repetitive stress.

Using these exercises will build up your shoulder strength and help fix your postural muscles to reduce your chances of developing an injury like a rotator cuff tear. As an added bonus, your fifth program will help you sculpt and define your arms.

Almost There! Workout Five

Let's Get Started!!!

Almost There! Workout Five

Protocol and Order:

- ♦ **(Warm Up)** Perform 7-10 minutes of cardio on the upright bike before you start your routine. Your heart rate should be between 100-120 bpm.

- ♦ **(Exercise)** Perform *three to four* circuits in order, keeping your heart rate between 150 and 170 bpm.

- ◆ **(Cardio)** Perform 10-15 minutes of cardio after your program on the upright bike with your heart rate between 140-160 bpm.
- ◆ **(Stretch)** Cool down using the stretches in this guide.

Duration: Week Five

Days per week: 2-3 (Leave 24 hours between sessions)

Exercise Reps: 10-12 or 12-15, depending on exercise

Load: Body weight or 45-55% 1 rep max

Circuits: 3-4

Rest interval: 15-30 seconds between exercises; 3-4 minutes between circuits

Equipment: Women: Two 5-8 lb dumbbells, two 8-10 lb dumbbells, two 10-12 lb dumbbells, and an 8 lb medicine ball

Men: Two 8-10 lb dumbbells, two 12-15 lb dumbbells, two 15-20 lb dumbbells, and a 10 lb medicine ball

Note: The last few reps on each exercise should be taxing. When you can comfortably perform the number of repetitions suggested, increase your weight.

Romanian Deadlift # 1

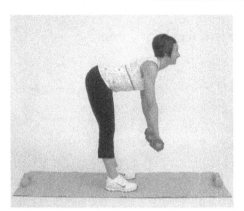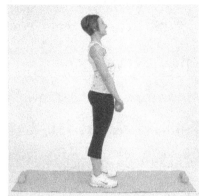

a. Start with your feet shoulder-width apart, bend over at the waist until your torso is parallel with the floor, and look up, keeping your head aligned with your spine.

b. Stick your butt up and out, keeping your chest up, and extend the dumbbells downward and in line with your shoulders (palms facing your legs).

c. While maintaining a flat back, gently thrust your hips forward while contracting your hamstrings and glutes until your body is upright with your hips in line with the rest of your spine. Return to the starting position and repeat.

Special Instructions:

Maintain only a slight bend in the knees and avoid rounding your back to prevent strain.

Perform: 10-12 repetitions
Women: 10-12 lb dumbbells (each hand)
Men: 15-20 lb dumbbells (each hand)

Overhead Asymmetrical Squat # 2

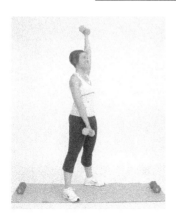 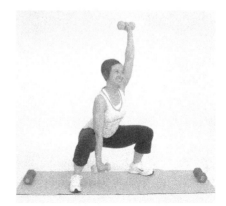

a. **(Part 1)** Stand with your feet slightly wider than shoulder-width apart. Turn your toes out so your hips and knees are in a straight line. Grab two dumbbells and drop one arm between your legs. Lift your chest up, and raise the other dumbbell straight up overhead with your palm facing outward.

b. **(Part 2)** Lower your body by bending at your knees while sticking your butt out, and continue squatting until your knees and hips are parallel. When squatting, keep your chest up and at a 45° angle to your hips while keeping the one dumbbell up overhead. Use your back, legs and core muscles to stabilize your body's position throughout the movement to avoid any rounding in your back.

c. **(Part 3)** While standing up, drive your hips forward until you can squeeze your butt cheeks together and until your hips and spine are in a neutral position. Complete all of your repetitions before switching sides and arms.

Perform: 10-12 repetitions
Women: 8-10 lb dumbbells (each hand)
Men: 12-15 lb dumbbells (each hand)

Medicine Ball Slam # 3

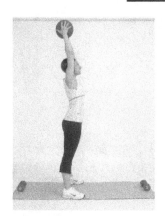 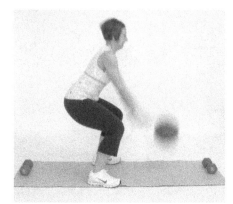

a. Stand with your feet slightly wider than shoulder-width apart and turn your toes out until your knees and hips are in a straight line.

b. Grab a medicine ball between your hands, pull it back behind your head, and hold it at arm's length overhead.

c. Forcefully throw the ball down on the ground as hard as possible while simultaneously squatting down. (Keep your arms straight while slamming the ball on the ground.)

d. Catch the ball as it bounces up from the ground. Stand up, return to the starting position, and repeat.

Special Instructions:

This is a timed exercise. Complete all of your reps in 20-25 seconds.

Perform: 12-15 repetitions
Women: 8 lb medicine ball
Men: 10 lb medicine ball

Bent Over Row # 4

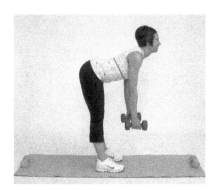 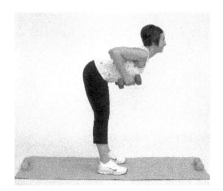

a. Bend over at the waist so your torso is parallel with the floor and your feet are shoulder-width apart.

b. Keep a slight bend in your knees (prevents lower back strain), stick your butt out, keep your chest up, and extend your arms downward with your palms facing each other.

c. While maintaining a flat back, raise your arms by bending at your elbows (while contracting your shoulders) until your shoulders are completely abducted.

d. Hold for a second and return until your arms are extended and your shoulders are stretched forward. Repeat.

Perform: 12-15 repetitions
Women: 8-12 lb dumbbells (each hand)
Men: 12-15 lb dumbbells (each hand)

Bent-Over Flye (Rear Delt Raise) # 5

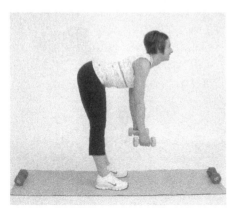 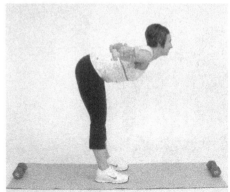

a. Grab the dumbbells in your hands with your palms toward each other. Stand with your feet shoulder-width apart. Bend forward at the waist until your torso is parallel to the floor, and extend your arms with the dumbbells downward.

b. Fully straighten your legs by sticking your butt up and out while driving up through your heels and lifting your chest up. If your hamstrings are too tight to fully straighten, it's okay to have a slight bend in your knees.

c. With your torso forward and stationary, inhale and lift the dumbbells straight to your sides until both arms are parallel to the floor. Make sure to keep a slight bend in your elbows. Return and repeat. Avoid swinging your torso or bringing your arms back instead of to your sides.

Perform: 12-15 repetitions
Women: 5-8 lb dumbbells (each hand)
Men: 8-10 lb dumbbells (each hand)

Upright Row # 6

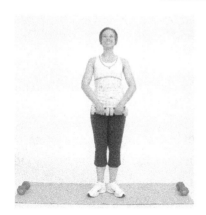 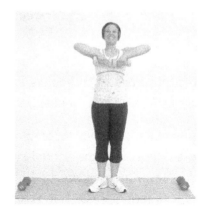

a. Stand with your back upright and feet together in a V-shape with legs and glutes contracted.

b. Extend your arms downward with wrists and elbows in a straight line and palms facing toward your body.

c. Raise the weights by bending your elbows upward. Let them travel along your body until your elbows are at a 90° angle and parallel with the floor.

d. Hold and return the dumbbells down your body the same way you brought them up. Repeat.

Special Instructions:

Keep your elbows elevated and above your wrists while you are lifting the weights.

Perform: 10-12 repetitions
Women: 8-10 lb dumbbells (each hand)
Men: 12-15 lb dumbbells (each hand)

Your Fifth Stretching Routine

Now that you're done with your workout, let's cool down!

What to Know

Your fifth workout program is designed to develop the strength and mobility of your upper body and shoulders to prevent injury.

By working to stretch these muscles out at the end of your routine, we can reduce any post-workout soreness that was created in your upper body and shoulders from these exercises while simultaneously improving the mobility and range of motion (ROM) in your upper body and shoulders.

Scalene Neck Stretch

- Grab your left arm behind your back with your right hand and pull down.

- Look straight ahead and lean your head to your right side like you're trying to touch your ear to your shoulder.

- Avoid lifting your shoulder while stretching.

Stretching Benefits:

Tight scalene muscles can cause nerve compression leading to dizziness, abnormal breathing patterns, migraine-like headaches, and feelings of nausea.

Perform: 2 sets of 1 repetition
Sides: Both
Hold stretch for 30 seconds.

Levator Scapulae Stretch

- Position your right arm behind your back if you're standing, or grab under a chair if you're sitting.

- Tip your head toward your left shoulder, and grab the back of your head with your left hand.

- Gently pull down on your head and avoid lifting your shoulder while you're stretching.

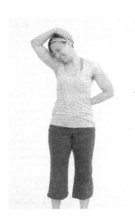

Stretching Benefits:

Tight levator scapulae muscles can make your neck become so tight that it is difficult to turn your neck because of the tension and pain.

Perform: 2 sets of 1 repetition
Sides: Both
Hold stretch for 30 seconds.

Kneeling Hip Flexor Stretch

- Kneel down on one knee with your other leg out in front.

- Place your hands on your knees.

- Lean forward keeping your chest and back upright until you can feel the stretch in the inside of your back leg.

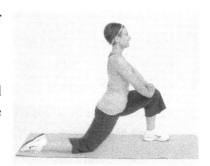

Stretching Benefits:

Tight hip flexor muscles can create stress to your groin, which can potentially cause a rupture or a tear to these muscles over time.

Perform: 2 sets of 1 repetition
Sides: Both
Hold stretch for 30 seconds.

Downward Dog (Calf) Stretch

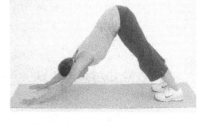

- Start on all fours with hands and knees shoulder-width apart.

- Breathe and push the palms of your hands into the floor. Drop your shoulders as you breathe.

- Slowly straighten your legs upward, push your pelvis toward the back wall, and lift your head. It's still okay to have a slight bend in your knees if you have tight calf and hamstring muscles.

Stretching Benefits:

Tight calf muscles can cause abnormal movement patterns in your ankles joints leading to ankle pain and shin splints.

Perform: 2 sets of 1 repetition
Hold stretch for 30 seconds.

Ball-Lying Chest Stretch

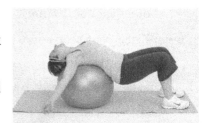

- Lie with your back on a balance ball.

- Roll down until your head and neck are fully supported.

- Relax your hips and let your arms fall out to your sides.

Stretching Benefits:

Tight chest muscles will cause your shoulders to round forward leading to upper back pain and to the dysfunction of your spinal joints.

Perform: 2 sets of 1 repetition
Hold stretch for 30 seconds.

Arm-Shoulder (Towel) Stretch

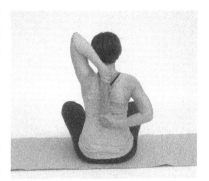

- Grab a hand towel and extend one hand down your back with your hand in line with your spine, pointing down.

- Use the other hand to reach behind your back to grab the towel.

- Gently pull down on the towel. Repeat by pulling up on the towel with the other hand.

Stretching Benefits:

Tight arm muscles can create stress to the tendons of your arms causing a tear.

Perform: 2 sets of 1 repetition
Sides: Both
Hold stretch for 30 seconds.

Chapter 6

visions of success

Moving Forward

It is extremely frustrating to gain weight after you've achieved success, especially when you have worked really hard to get your new body, and you've started to feel like this time, it's for real.

Over the past five weeks, you have being learning new skills and habits that have allowed you to lose weight. Now that we are getting close to the end of your body challenge, I want to give you some additional strategies you can use to help maintain your weight loss long term and avoid a rebound.

1. **You must be fully committed with a strong desire to maintain long-term change outside of your immediate weight-loss goals.**

I always tell my clients during our first session together that weight loss is about dedicating yourself to creating positive and productive habits that you can sustain long term. You must be passionate about your desire to change, and you must be consistent with your efforts to achieve your goals.

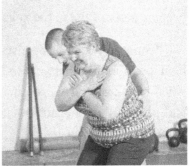

I have seen many clients who were talented and successful in other areas of their lives fail to maintain their weight loss. The reason they failed is that weight loss was their immediate goal and not their long-term plan.

An immediate goal such as getting in shape for a wedding, looking good at the beach, or getting ready for a reunion might be a good motivator to begin your weight-loss journey, but without a personal commitment to losing weight and changing your life outside of these immediate short-term goals, you will have difficulties maintaining your results.

How to Overcome:

The most successful clients I have worked with are the ones who come to me primarily to improve their health. They are the clients who've just had their yearly visit to the doctor and were told to reduce their body fat and cholesterol levels due to major risk factors. I've also had clients come to me because they have a family history of heart disease and have recently had a close family member suffer from heart attack.

The reason that these clients are successful is that they have a very powerful internal reason for wanting to maintain their success long after they achieved their immediate weight-loss goals.

During this last week of your body challenge, do some brainstorming, and list some enduring sources of personal motivation that can keep you going once you are finished with your **Six-Week Body Challenge**.

2.   Surround yourself with other people who also want to lose weight.

I have seen clients fail to maintain their weight loss because they have become susceptible to the negative influences of well-meaning people.

People in your life who struggle with their own weight-loss journeys may be uncomfortable that you are attempting to succeed at your goals, especially when they aren't. This is a difficult situation, as these people can feel jealous and project their negativity onto you. Without really meaning to, they may derail you from succeeding.

Other people in your life may not have the same goals and desires as you do, so they don't understand why you are pushing yourself so hard. Although they really care about you, they want to eat and do whatever they want. They may eat junk food around you, or they may want you to join their social activities, like going out for pizza and beer. This is a difficult situation, as you care for these people even though they don't share your interest in being healthy.

Unfortunately, you may also come across cynics who are angry at life. These are the worst kinds of people to be around. They like to complain about everything from their bosses to their favorite sports teams, and if you spend any time around them, you end up getting caught in their whirlpools of negative activity. These people are simply mad at life and sincerely enjoy bringing others down with them. They will find all kinds of different reasons to make you feel bad about yourself and your desire to be healthy.

Being around critical people is a dangerous thing when you're developing new habits. If you lose the sincere belief that you deserve to be successful, you will want to give up. And then, you will.

How to Overcome:

Believe in yourself and your abilities, and make it a habit to surround yourself with people that will motivate you to take action.

Find a friend or a gym buddy who can exercise with you, and create a schedule that allows you to go to the gym together on a regular basis. This will make it much easier for you to stay motivated and push yourself. The accountability of a workout partner who is relying on you to show up is an extremely powerful motivator. You will also find that you'll get a much more intense workout exercising with a buddy than on your own because your buddy won't let you slack off.

You can become part of a group at work that goes for walks during lunch breaks or wants to the gym after work. You can also join a local sports team to be around other like-minded people – just make sure that the emphasis isn't solely on going out drinking afterward!

I also really like the idea of using a weight-loss support group, like Weight Watchers, or an online group if you don't have access to something similar in your area. These groups give you a chance to share your experiences and struggles with the others who are going through the same thing. It also gives you freedom to express yourself without the fear of being judged. This type of support can make all the difference in your ability to succeed.

3.   Create a sustainable game plan to lose weight, and maintain it.

Being successful on your own is about creating a realistic game plan for how much weight you either want to lose or maintain each week and month.

When coming up with your game plan, make sure that your expectations are reasonable for what you can achieve based on your weekly schedule, and remember not to compare yourself to others.

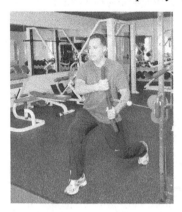

It is important to realize that some individuals can lose weight faster than others due to their genetic predispositions, and younger adults may have an easier time losing weight because their cells divide more often, giving them a higher metabolic rate. (The metabolic rate of older adults, however, can be increased through use of consistent strength training over a period of two to three months.)

Don't be fooled by weight-loss products that make any of the following false promises:

- You will lose weight without diet and exercise.
- You will lose weight no matter how much food you eat.
- You will lose 30 pounds in 30 days (or similar).
- You will permanently lose weight by blocking the absorption of fat and calories.

A realistic game plan recognizes that weight loss is about consistent, healthy patterns and that real, sustainable results are not achieved overnight.

How to Overcome:

When designing your game plan, start by creating smaller, more attainable goals. Succeeding in these smaller initial goals will help feed your need to achieve bigger goals while also making you feel really good about yourself. (For more information about goal setting, reference the SMART system described in the conclusion.)

Remember that the average fat loss for most people is also about one to two pounds a week. While you may see a bigger drop in the first few weeks of any new program, one to two pounds a week is an extremely fast pace. That works out to a consistent fat loss of two pounds a week, eight pounds a month, and over one hundred pounds a year!

Remember that your success is about being consistent, being persistent, and being able to give your program time to work for you.

4. Forgive yourself for your mistakes, and start over right now!

There will always be temptations like junk food at home or the office, parties, and social gatherings with friends and family. Food is a huge part of how we socialize in America, but the food we eat isn't always the problem. Rather, it's the "all or nothing" attitude that many of us have developed when it comes to diet and exercise.

We all make mistakes, and if you are going to be successful, you need to be able to forgive yourself. If not, you can develop terrible feelings of guilt and anxiety over the mistakes that you've made in the past. These feelings can lead you to stop exercising and splurge even more. This can become a vicious cycle where you eventually feel so frustrated that you simply want to quit altogether.

This is also the problem with strict diets. They don't take into account your likes or dislikes, and they require you to change everything overnight. This does not work for many people because these changes are only temporary. If you have no intention of making these changes habitual, you will gain back any weight you have lost as soon as you are done dieting.

How to Overcome:

Rather than criticizing yourself every time you mess up, stop in that moment and use your mistakes as feedback. After all, you probably didn't intentionally set out to screw up in the first place.

Also, allow yourself time to make the more gradual changes that you know you can incorporate into your lifestyle. It is much easier to take your time to figure out a process that works for you rather than to shotgun a whole bunch of things at once. This gives you the time you need to know which changes are sustainable and appropriate for what you are trying to achieve.

Remember to have fun while you are creating your own game plan, and know that you deserve to be successful. I believe in you!

H2 Oh My!

Water and Exercise Nutrition

Water

Properly hydrating yourself for exercise is essential if you want to be successful, especially as your intensity level goes up. When you exercise at a higher intensity, you are able to burn more calories in the same period of time and lose weight faster. However, as your intensity level increases, you sweat more, and you'll need more water to balance your electrolyte levels and keep cool.

The Break Down

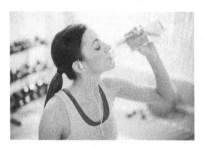 The adult body is mainly composed of water, and when you exercise, your internal body temperature rises as your muscles produce energy. This causes you to sweat as a means of keeping cool. The more intense your exercise, the more you'll sweat. The key to staying well-hydrated when you exercise is to drink water before, during and after your workout. If you wait to drink water until you are thirsty, your body will already be in the early stages of dehydration, and it will become difficult for you to complete your exercise routine. Some of the signs and symptoms of dehydration include a headache, a rapid or an irregular heartbeat, dizziness, dry-mouth, muscle cramping and pre-mature fatigue. Once you start to feel fatigue, your body slows down, and your chances for injury increase because your muscles have a tougher time responding to the demands of your workout. So, how do you know if you are drinking enough water to avoid becoming dehydrated?

How Much Water Do You Need?

The average adult should drink half of his or her body weight in fluid ounces every day to stay hydrated. For example, if you're a male who weighs

160 pounds, you will need to consume 80 fluid ounces (fl oz) or roughly ten (8oz) glasses of water every day to keep your body running efficiently. However, you will need more water than that on the days you exercise. Try the following schedule for drinking water on those days in addition to your regular water consumption:

Hydrating before you exercise:

- Drink 1-2 glasses of water an hour or two hours before you exercise and then drink another glass 30 minutes before your work out.

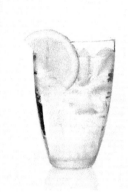

Hydrating while you are exercising:

- Drink one glass of water for every 20 to 30 minutes of exercise.

Hydrating after you exercise:

- Weigh yourself before and after your workout, and drink 1-2 glasses of water for every pound of water weight that you lost.

Sports drinks are a good substitute for plain water during exercise as they contain electrolytes that are often lost during exercise. This helps prevent muscle cramping afterward. Sports drink can also increase your intestines' ability to absorb water. However, you need to be careful when using sports drinks. Many sports drinks contain excessive amounts of calories in the form of sugar, and the heavy use of sports drinks can cause unwanted weight gain.

A good substitute for a sports drink is a fresh glass of orange juice. Fresh orange juice contains less sugar than processed and frozen orange juices, and your body needs the carbohydrates in the orange juice to help with muscle recovery. Orange juice also contains large amounts potassium and other electrolytes needed to maintain a proper amount of fluid within your body. However, make sure that you are not consuming too much, as it can also lead to unwanted weight gain.

Hydration Tips

Here are a few tips to help you drink more water throughout the day:

1. Carry a bottle of water with you wherever you go. Water is like many other things: if it is out of sight, it is out of mind. By carrying a bottle of purified water with you wherever you go, you increase your ability to consume more water throughout the day. Having to refill your bottle at work will also give you a reason to get up and move around, especially if you have a desk job. Since sitting for extended periods of time will cause muscle soreness and tension, periodically moving around helps reduce muscle tension, specifically in your neck, shoulders, and low back.

2. Lemon, orange and lime wedges are great for adding flavor to water. They also add extra vitamin C to your water and help reduce your cravings for flavored beverages, which will also help you lose weight. The average soda contains 150 calories, most of which are refined sugars.

3. Low-calorie options like Crystal Light's "Pure" brand packets are also great. They add a lot of flavor to your water, each packet is low in calories, and they come in several varieties. The "Pure" line also adds a small amount of electrolytes in each packet, and each packet uses Truvia™ as a sweetener instead of processed and refined sugars, reducing the amount of calories you are consuming per serving. (Truvia™ is a stevia based sweetener.)

Your Sixth Menu

Menu Benefits (Water and Fiber)

Getting plenty of water and fiber in your diet will help to regulate your blood sugar levels, which is important in avoiding diabetes. Increasing your fiber intake can also reduce your risk of heart disease and gastrointestinal problems like constipation. Fiber absorbs large amounts of water your GI tract, making it easier for your intestines to pass waste.

This week's menu is full of fresh fruits and vegetables, adding lots of extra water and fiber into your diet. It also includes a homemade Santa Fe Chicken Chili that is anything but ordinary!

Notes on This Week's Menu

The same rules apply for changing the order of your meals this week. Remember that this is the last week of your body challenge, so now is the perfect time to record your weight, to take your measurements, and to take follow-up pictures before you send me your progress report!

Your breakfast this week is intended to be made into an enjoyable chocolate and peanut butter smoothie. The bread, pizza sauce, and cheese in your dinner menu are meant to be made into cheesy bread to go with your chicken chili. Simply heat your oven to 450°, place your bread on an oven-safe cooking pan, spread your pizza sauce evenly, layer your half a slice of cheese on top, and cook until done. Enjoy!

Special Entrée of the Week

Santa Fe Chicken Chili combines fire roasted tomatoes with a special three-bean blend, farm-fresh chicken, bold red and yellow peppers and onions, and a special blend of seasonings simmered to perfection to give you amazing homemade chili.

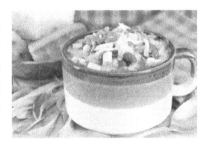

This recipe is available for only $0.99 at:
CustomWorkoutVideos.com/catalog/index.php

Women's Menu: Week Six

Breakfast	Serving Size	Calories	Grams Protein Carbs, Fat	Comments
Creamy Peanut Butter	1 tbsp (0.5oz)	100 cal	4g protein, 3.5g carbs, 8g fat	based on Natural Creamy Jif
Chocolate Almond Milk	1 cup (8oz)	105 cal	1.5g protein, 18g carbs, 3g fat	based on Blue Diamond brand milk
Pineapple Greek Yogurt	1 cup (6oz)	140 cal	14g protein, 20g carbs, 0g fat	based on no-fat Chobani brand yogurt
Banana	1 small (3.6oz)	90 cal	1g protein, 23g carbs, 0.5g fat	based on an average organic brand
Dark Chocolate Powder	2 tbsp (0.4oz)	40 cal	2g protein, 6g carbs, 1g fat	based on Hershey's Dark Chocolate Powder

Snacks	Serving Size	Calories	Grams Protein Carbs, Fat	Comments
Chocolate Fudge Brownie	1 bar	90 cal	1g protein, 18g carbs, 3g fat	based on Fiber One Brand

Lunch	Serving Size	Calories	Grams Protein Carbs, Fat	Comments
Rosemary Olive Oil Bread	1 slice (1.4oz)	100 cal	4g protein, 20g carbs, 1g fat	based on Rudi's Organic (can be traded for wheat)
Deli Meat Smoked Turkey or Roast Beef	1 serving (2oz)	60 cal	12g protein, 0g carbs, 3g fat	based on Applegate Farms deli meat

Sharp Cheddar or Swiss Cheese Slice	1 slice (1oz)	110 cal	7g protein, 0g carbs, 9g fat	based on Trader Joes sharp cheddar cheese
Butterhead Lettuce	2 slices (0.4oz)	<1cal	0g protein, <1g carbs, 0g fat	based on an average organic brand
Roma Tomatoes	4 slices (2.8oz)	14 cal	<1g protein, 3g carbs, 0g fat	based on an average organic brand
Yellow Mustard	1-2 tsp (0.2oz)	0 cal	0g protein, <1g carbs, 0g fat	based on French's classic yellow mustard

Snacks	Serving Size	Calories	Grams Protein Carbs, Fat	Comments
Orange or Apple	1 small (3.4oz)	50 cal	1g protein, 11.5g carbs, 0g fat	based on an average organic brand

Dinner	Serving Size	Calories	Grams Protein Carbs, Fat	Comments
*Santa Fe Chicken Chili	1 serving (12.5oz)	290 cal	33g protein, 32g carbs, 3g fat	Custom Workout Videos.com brand
Rosemary Olive Oil Bread	1 slice (1.4oz)	100 cal	4g protein, 20g carbs, 1g fat	based on Rudi's Organic (can be changed for wheat)
Pizza Sauce	0.25 cup (2oz)	65 cal	2g protein, 9g carbs, 2.5g fat	based on Eden Organic Pizza Sauce
Sharp Cheddar or Colby Jack Cheese Slice	0.5 slice (0.5oz)	55 cal	3.5g protein, 0g carbs, 4.5g fat	based on Trader Joes sharp cheddar cheese

Men's Menu: Week Six

Breakfast	Serving Size	Calories	Grams Protein Carbs, Fat	Comments
Creamy Peanut Butter	2 tbsp (1oz)	200 cal	8g protein, 7g carbs, 16g fat	based on Natural Creamy Jif
Chocolate Almond Milk	1 cup (8oz)	105 cal	1.5g protein, 18g carbs, 3g fat	based on Blue Diamond brand milk
Pineapple Greek Yogurt	1 cup (6oz)	140 cal	14g protein, 20g carbs, 0g fat	based on no-fat Chobani brand yogurt
Banana	1 medium (4.2oz)	120 cal	1g protein, 27g carbs, 0.5g fat	based on an average organic brand
Dark Chocolate Powder	1 tbsp (0.2oz)	20 cal	1g protein, 3g carbs, 0.5g fat	based on Hershey's Dark Chocolate Powder

Snacks	Serving Size	Calories	Grams Protein Carbs, Fat	Comments
Raspberry Greek Yogurt	1 cup (6oz)	140 cal	14g protein, 20g carbs, 0g fat	based on no-fat Chobani brand yogurt
Blueberries	0.5 cup (2.5oz)	41 cal	0.5g protein, 11g carbs, 0g fat	based on an average organic brand

Lunch	Serving Size	Calories	Grams Protein Carbs, Fat	Comments
Rosemary Olive Oil Bread	2 slices (2.8oz)	200 cal	8g protein, 40g carbs, 2g fat	based on Rudi's Organic (can be changed for wheat bread)

Deli Meat Smoked Turkey or Roast Beef	1 serving (2oz)	60 cal	12g protein, 0g carbs, 3g fat	based on Applegate Farms deli meat
Sharp Cheddar or Swiss Cheese Slice	1 slice (1oz)	110 cal	7g protein, 0g carbs, 9g fat	based on Trader Joes sharp cheddar cheese
Butterhead Lettuce	2 slices (0.4oz)	<1cal	0g protein, <1g carbs, 0g fat	based on an average organic brand
Roma Tomatoes	4 slices (2.8oz)	14 cal	<1g protein, 3g carbs, 0g fat	based on an average organic brand
Yellow Mustard	1-2 tsp (0.2oz)	0 cal	0g protein, <1g carbs, 0g fat	based on French's classic yellow mustard

Snacks	Serving Size	Calories	Grams Protein Carbs, Fat	Comments
Chocolate Fudge Brownie	1 bar	90 cal	1g protein, 18g carbs, 3g fat	based on Fiber One Brand
Orange or Apple	1 small (3.4oz)	50 cal	1g protein, 11.5g carbs, 0g fat	based on an average organic brand

Dinner	Serving Size	Calories	Grams Protein Carbs, Fat	Comments
*Santa Fe Chicken Chili	1 serving (12.5oz)	290 cal	33g protein, 32g carbs, 3g fat	Custom Workout Videos.com brand
Rosemary Olive Oil Bread	1 slice (1.4oz)	100 cal	4g protein, 20g carbs, 1g fat	based on Rudi's Organic (can be changed for wheat)

Pizza Sauce	0.25 cup (2oz)	65 cal	2g protein, 9g carbs, 2.5g fat	based on Eden Organic Pizza Sauce
Sharp Cheddar or Colby Jack Cheese Slice	0.5 slice (0.5oz)	55 cal	3.5g protein, 0g carbs, 4.5g fat	based on Trader Joes sharp cheddar cheese

Your Sixth Cardio Plan

Modifications and Benefits

Benefits

Your sixth cardiovascular program is designed to help you blast through fitness plateaus with your cardiovascular training. This will allow you to accomplish even more physically demanding tasks with fewer problems, which will be extremely important as you are now living a more active lifestyle and preparing to move on into the future.

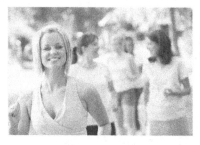

Fitness plateaus happen to everyone. Our bodies are designed to adapt to the physical demands we place upon them—especially repetitive ones. This is why you can't do the same workout routine everyday and see long-term results. This applies as much to your cardio routine as it does to your workout routine, and once you hit a plateau, it will become harder and harder to build muscle and lose weight. For this reason, you need to make regular changes to your fitness routines.

In order to keep you from dropping into a fitness plateau, we'll be changing your cardio routine again this week. This is why I've been changing your cardio and workout routines throughout this guide. These changes will also help you develop different parts of your body.

As you move forward on your own, here are five different things that you can do to avoid reaching a plateau:

1. Increase the frequency of your workouts by adding in one extra session a week. Don't work out more than 4-5 days a week, however, or you can end up overtraining, which can cause injury.

2. Increase your intensity by increasing speed, resistance or the incline of your machine. This is one of the easiest ways to push through a plateau. You can also increase your duration by increasing the amount of time you spend doing your cardio by five or ten minutes.

3. Change the machines or types of cardio you do on a regular basis. Something as small as changing activities will work the body in a whole new way and help you achieve better results, even if the intensity is the same.

4. Do interval training. Interval training involves alternating between higher and lower intensities. For an example on how to set up your cardio program with intervals, see the cardio modifications recommended for your programs in chapters three and four.

Remember that change is good. Now, let's make that push towards the finish line!

Your Sixth Cardio Program

Warm Up (7-10 min) Perform 7-10 minutes of light cardio by walking on the treadmill before you engage in your workout routine. Your heart rate should be between 100-120 bpm—about 50-55% of your maximum heart rate. This zone will warm your body up and get you ready for action.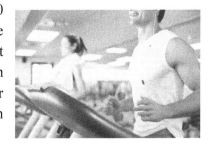

Cardio: End of Program (10-15 min) Do 10-15 minutes of cardio by running on the treadmill after your program. This is week six, so let's make sure to get your heart rate up between 160-180 bpm.

This training zone is closer to 75-85% of your maximum heart rate, and this intensity will help build your circulatory system. This will prepare your body for the higher intensities needed to strengthen your circulatory system so that you can push yourself during your circuit training program.

Remember, when you're training at this intensity you'll be breathing fairly heavily, and you're not going to be speaking in sentences. You will be struggling to speak altogether and will only gasp out single words at a time. Use these physiological cues to reinforce when you are training within the right zone.

This is the culmination of everything that you have been working for over the last six weeks. Push yourself hard because you are ready to cross the finish line. I am really proud of you for sticking in there and getting the job done! Yeah!!!

Program Modifications

Your level of cardiovascular conditioning should be dramatically changing for the better, so any program modifications required should be limited. If you still require some modifications to your cardio program, no problem. However, I am going to ask you to push yourself hard. This is week six, and I want you to finish strong!

If needed, alternate your intensity on the treadmill between the lower intensity of last week (140-160bpm) and the higher intensity of this week (160-180bpm). Alternate the intensities by going for one minute at the higher intensity and then for two minutes at the lower intensity until done. Remember, to slow down long enough for the feeling to pass if you get dizzy, lightheaded or are unable to catch your breath.

Also, if you don't have access to a treadmill, here are some suggestions:

1. Go to your local community center or YMCA. They should have a treadmill you can use along with some space and exercise equipment you can use for your exercise routine afterward. (Community centers also tend to cost very little to use for the day and usually have running tracks even if they don't have a treadmill.)

2. Go for a run or jog outside before your workout. Most community parks have a running track that you can use, especially if you don't have any running trails or paths nearby. If it's cold outside, buy a jump rope, and do your cardio at home. It should be easy to get your heart rate up from jumping rope. Make sure to push yourself hard—no excuses. This is your last week!

Way to Go! Workout Six

What to Know

Ah, week six! This is the culmination of everything that you have been working for over the last several weeks. I am more than a little ecstatic.

This week's program has so many different training elements combined into one heck of a calorie-busting workout that I don't know where to begin! So let's touch on the major two.

The purpose of combining these elements into one program is to take the strength that you have been building over the last several weeks and convert it into functional power to improve your reflex action and your overall strength. To do this, I'm using a training technique called "contrast system training." With the elements of contrast system training in your program design, you'll have exercises that range from a heavier weight (Upright Row) immediately to another exercise that consists of little-to-no weight (Medicine Ball Slam). By using this method of exercise within your circuit training routine, your central nervous system will develop a faster muscle-response time by increasing the firing rate of your nerves. To best accomplish this, you'll need to remember that these specifically marked exercises are timed, and you will need to complete all of the repetitions for these exercises in 20 to 25 seconds. In doing so, we'll create some really nice and immediate strength gains for your body, especially if you're not used to this type of workout.

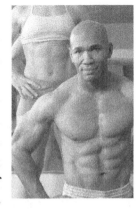

The other training element that I'm adding into your program is called "complex system training." This program utilizes exercises that work opposite muscles groups. For example, you'll have one exercise that is designed to work your arms and legs (Overhead Squat), and then you'll have another exercise that is designed to work your shoulders and back (Bent-Over Flye). This training element is great because it not only increases the amount of muscles that you're using in one workout to help you burn fat, but it also increases the amount of multi-planar, multi-directional stress that is placed your joints for increased stability and function (similar to week three).

Thus, I would say that week six is my favorite program. I hope you enjoy this program as much as I enjoyed designing it for you. I want you to feel the tremendous power and strength in who you are and what you can accomplish!

Way to Go! Workout Six

Let's Get Started!!!

Way to Go! Workout Six

Protocol and Order:

- ◆ **(Warm Up)** Walk for 7-10 minutes on the treadmill before you start your routine, keeping your heart rate between 100-120 bpm.

- ◆ **(Exercise)** Perform *three to four* circuits in order, keeping your heart rate between 150-170 bpm.

- ◆ **(Cardio)** Perform 10-15 minutes of cardio by running on the treadmill after your program with your heart rate between 160-180 bpm.

- ◆ **(Stretch)** Cool down using the stretches in this guide.

Duration: Week Six

Days per week: 2-3 (Leave 24 hours between sessions)

Exercise Reps: 10-12, 12-15, 15-20, depending on exercise

Load: Body weight or 55-65% 1 rep max

Circuits: 3-4

Rest interval: 15-30 seconds between exercises; 4-5 minutes between circuits

Equipment: Women: 12-15 lb body bar, two 8-10 lb dumbbells, two 12-15 lb dumbbells, and an 8 lb medicine ball

Men: 15-18 lb body bar, two 10-12 lb dumbbells, two 12-15 lb dumbbells, two 15-20 lb dumbbells, and a 10 lb medicine ball

Note: The last few reps on each exercise should be taxing. When you can comfortably perform the number of repetitions suggested, increase your weight.

Lateral Lunge # 1

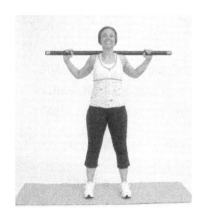
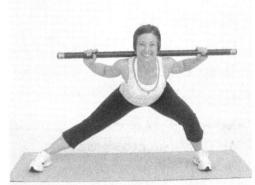

a. **(Part 1)** Stand upright with your feet slightly wider than shoulder-width apart. Tighten your upper back by pinching your shoulder blades together, and rest the bar on the muscles of your upper back just below the bone at the top of your shoulder blades. Your hands should be shoulder-width apart with your palms out and your elbows back. This will protect your elbows from injuries. (The bar should remain horizontal throughout the exercise.)

b. **(Part 2)** Lunge your body laterally to one side while moving your hips in the same direction, straightening out your supporting leg as you do. Land by planting onto your lunging foot, then by leaning back onto your heel.

c. Make sure to lunge into a wide stance. This will allow you adequate room to move your hips backward while keeping your lunging knee behind your toes to prevent knee strain.

d. **(Part 3)** The supporting leg should remain extended as you lower your body by bending at your knees while sticking your butt out. Continue to lower your body until the knee and hip of your lunging leg are parallel to one another. Keep your chest up and at a 45° angle to your hips when squatting. This is to avoid any rounding in the back, which can cause you lower back pain.

e. **(Part 4)** Once your full range of motion has been attained, return to the starting position by driving your hips upward and forward until your hips are aligned in a neutral position with your spine. The back should remain flat throughout the movement with your chest up. Return and repeat all repetitions to one side before switching.

Special Instructions:

Before you begin performing this exercise dynamically by lunging side-to-side, practice this exercise by squatting in the ending position, with one leg straight, eight to ten times on each side to get familiar with the movement.

Perform: 10-12 repetitions (each side) – hands in back squat position
Women: 12-15 lb body bar
Men: 15-18 lb body bar

Modified (Sumo Squat) Deadlift # 2

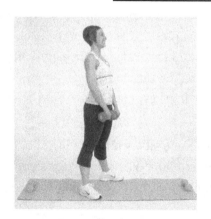 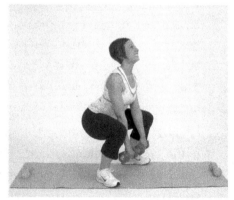

a. **(Part 1)** Stand with your feet slightly wider than shoulder-width apart, and turn your toes out until your knees are in line with your hips. Squat down by sticking your butt out while elevating your chest to avoid rounding your back. (Rounding your back can cause injury.)

b. As you bend down, hold the dumbbells down between your legs. letting your arms move along the inside of your legs. Continue to squat down until the points of your elbows touch the inside of your thighs.

c. **(Part 2)** While keeping your chest elevated, exhale and gently thrust your hips forward while contracting your hamstrings and glutes until your body is upright. Keep your back flat as you lift off the floor and extend through the heels. Repeat.

Perform: 12-15 repetitions
Women: 12-15 lb dumbbells (each hand)
Men: 15-20 lb dumbbells (each hand)

Squat Jumps # 3

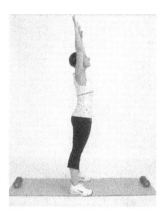
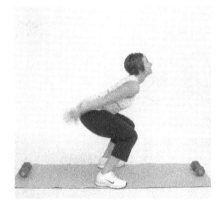
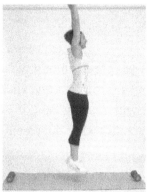

a. Stand with your feet shoulder-width apart and arms straight up overhead. Lower yourself into a squatted position, then, immediately jump up as high as you can, swinging your arms up overhead, and look up. This will help straighten your body and move your hips forward to help you maximize your jump and the effects of the exercise.

b.   Softly land on the balls of your feet, then on your heels, while bringing your arms back and finish in a squat position. Repeat immediately. (Delaying your next jump will limit the effects of the exercise.)

Special Instructions:

This is a timed exercise. Complete all of your reps in 20-25 seconds.

Perform: 15-20 repetitions
Women: Bodyweight
Men: Bodyweight

Overhead Squat # 4

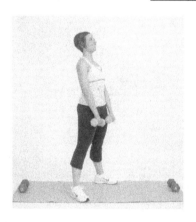 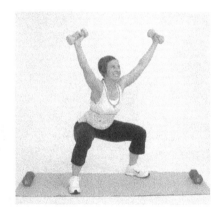

a.   **(Part 1)** Stand with your feet slightly wider than shoulder-width apart and turn your toes out so your hips and knees are in a straight line. Grab two dumbbells and, with a slight bend in your elbows, drop your arms down by your knees with your palms facing your legs.

b.   **(Part 2)** Lower your body by bending at your knees while sticking your butt out, and lower your body until your knees and hips are parallel. Keep your chest up and at a 45° angle to your hips when squatting.

c.   While squatting, raise both dumbbells up and back until you can squeeze your shoulder blades together. Use your legs, your back and the rest of your core muscles to stabilize your body position.

d.   **(Part 3)** While standing, drive your hips forward until you can squeeze your butt cheeks together and until your back is straight. Drop the dumbbells. Repeat.

Perform: 12-15 repetitions
Women: 8-10 lb dumbbells (each hand)
Men: 12-15 lb dumbbells (each hand)

Medicine Ball Slam # 5

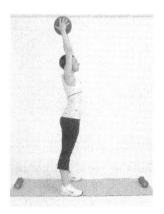 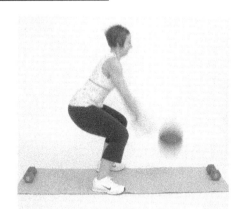

a. Stand with your feet slightly wider than shoulder-width apart and turn your toes out until your knees and hips are in a straight line.

b. Grab the medicine ball between your hands, pull it back behind your head, and hold it at arm's length overhead.

c. Forcefully throw the ball down on the ground as hard as possible while squatting.

d. Keep your arms straight while slamming the ball on the ground, and catch the ball as it bounces up. Stand up, return to starting position, and repeat.

Special Instructions:

This is a timed exercise. Complete all of your reps in 20-25 seconds.

Perform: 15-20 repetitions
Women: 8 lb medicine ball
Men: 10 lb medicine ball

Bent-Over Flye (Rear Delt Raise) # 6

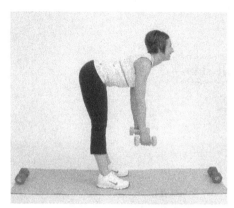 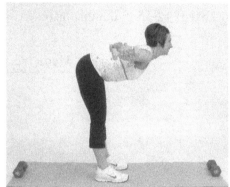

a. Grab the dumbbells with your palms facing each other. Stand with your feet shoulder-width apart. Bend forward at the waist until your torso is parallel to the floor, and extend your dumbbells downward.

b. Fully straighten your legs by sticking your butt up and out while driving up through your heels. Lift your chest up. If your hamstrings are too tight to fully straighten, it's okay to have a slight bend in your knees.

c. With your torso forward and stationary, exhale and lift the dumbbells straight to your sides until both arms are parallel to the floor, keeping a slight bend in your elbows. Avoid swinging your torso or bringing your arms back instead of to your sides. Return and repeat.

Perform: 10-12 repetitions
Women: 8-10 lb dumbbells (each hand)
Men: 10-12 lb dumbbells (each hand)

Your Sixth Stretching Routine

Now that you're done with your workout, let's cool down!

What to Know

Your sixth exercise routine is designed to convert the strength that you've been building into functional strength and power to improve your reflexes.

To help offset any soreness that you might experience at the end of your workout; this routine will help promote blood flow and stretch out your entire body.

Scalene Neck Stretch

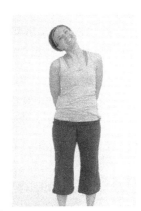

- Grab your left arm behind your back with your right hand and pull down.

- Look straight ahead and lean your head to your right side like you're trying to touch your ear to your shoulder.

- Avoid lifting your shoulder while stretching.

Stretching Benefits:

Tight scalene muscles are a common source of headaches and can send pain to the front of your chest, causing false angina.

Perform: 2 sets of 1 repetition
Sides: Both
Hold stretch for 30 seconds.

Levator Scapulae Stretch

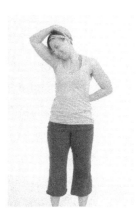

- Position your right arm behind your back if you're standing or grab underneath a chair if you're sitting.

- Tip your head toward your left shoulder and grab the back of your head with your left hand.

- Gently pull down on your head, and avoid lifting your shoulder while you're stretching.

Stretching Benefits:

Tight levator scapulae muscles can cause numbness, tingling, or a feeling of burning that extends over the back of your head as well as eye pain and blurred vision.

Perform: 2 sets of 1 repetition
Sides: Both
Hold stretch for 30 seconds.

get skinny!

Standing Side Stretch

- Stand with your legs wide apart with your right leg out in front.

- Point your right toes straight forward and your left toes out until your feet make a T-shape.

- Twist and place your right elbow on your thigh, straighten your left arm up, and stretch toward the opposite wall.

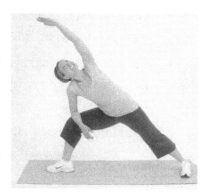

Stretching Benefits:

Tight latissimus dorsi muscles can make it hard for your ribs to expand during respiration, making breathing difficult.

Perform: 2 sets of 1 repetition
Sides: Both
Hold stretch for 30 Seconds.

Downward Dog (Calf) Stretch

- Start on all fours with hands and knees shoulder-width apart.

- Breathe and push the palms of your hands into the floor. Drop your shoulders as you breathe.

- Slowly straighten your legs upward, push your pelvis towards the back wall, and lift your head up.

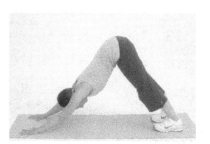

Stretching Benefits:

Tight calf muscles can restrict blood flow causing blood pooling and clotting in your extremities.

Perform: 2 sets of 1 repetition
Hold exercise for 30 seconds.

Hamstring Stretch

- Keep your back upright.
- Straighten one leg while tucking the other in.
- Lean forward with your back upright until you are comfortably stretching the backside of your leg.

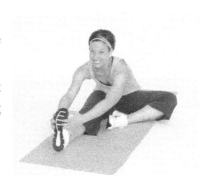

Stretching Benefits:

Tight hamstring muscles can cause back pain by pulling your pelvis out of its normal alignment.

Perform: 2 sets of 1 repetition
Sides: Both
Hold exercise for 30 seconds.

Pigeon Pose (Glute) Stretch

- Start on your hands and knees. Bend one leg out in front of you on the floor.
- Place the other leg straight out behind you.
- Use your arms to slowly push your torso upright until you feel the stretch in the gluteal side of your bent leg.

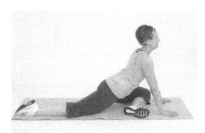

Stretching Benefits:

Tight gluteal muscles can put pressure on your sacroiliac (SI) joint, leading to lower back pain and inflammation.

Perform: 2 sets of 1 repetition
Hold exercise for 30 seconds.

Conclusion

Congratulations!!! You did it!

This **Six-Week Body Challenge** has all been about helping you create a better quality of life by becoming more physically fit. It has been an extreme pleasure for me to have worked with you during these last six weeks. Thank you for allowing me to be a part of your own personal fitness journey!

To help support you as you move forward, I have created a free bonus workout program just for you, along with a free bonus recipe to go along with your exercise program.

I want to invite you to sign up for my Facebook fan page (facebook. com/scottschmaltz.fanpage) as well as my email newsletter at: *www. CustomWorkoutVideos.com*. This will allow me to stay in touch with you as you progress. After you sign up, send me an email at: scott@customworkoutvideos. com and I'll send your free bonus workout program and recipe!

In the meantime, I would like to help you by breaking down a system that I personally use for goal-setting: the Be SMART system. As I mentioned in week six of your program, being successful on your own is about creating a realistic game plan for how much weight you either want to lose or maintain each week and each month.

The Be SMART system stands for setting Specific, Measurable, Action-Oriented, Realistic and Timed goals to achieve success.

Specific: "Wanting to stay in shape" is not specific enough. Spend time creating objectives that will help you stay in shape, like doing 30 minutes of moderate-intensity cardio a minimum of three to four days a week. If you have a busy schedule, then a specific goal could be to do some form of physical activity, like resistance training, a minimum of two to three times per week while watching your favorite television show. (For quick videos on exercises that you can do in front of the television, visit my website at: *www. CustomWorkoutVideos.com*, and check out the links under "Free Workouts.")

It is also extremely important that you set goals for your food intake. A great goal can be to consume only one small portion of your favorite dessert at family gatherings. Another could be to limit your alcohol consumption to only one or two drinks while there. It is very easy to "fall off the wagon" if you don't have a specific strategy set for family get-togethers. (This strategy is also my preferred method for going out to eat with friends and family.) Make a game plan about what you are or are not going to eat and drink before you get there, and then stick to it!

Measurable: When setting goals, it's important to have some system of measuring and rewarding yourself for success. Otherwise, how will you know if you are doing well?

You can write down your successes to help keep you motivated. A good example can be to give yourself a smiley face on the calendar every time you get to the gym and work out during the week. That way, if you don't see a lot of smiley faces, you know you'd better get to work.

Also, make sure to write a two or three word notation on the calendar next to your smiley face like, "tired, exercised anyway." This will not only help you remember why you received the smiley face in the first place, but it will also help reinforce the new and positive habits that you're trying to create. It will also help keep you focused on your successes rather than your failures, which will boost your motivation and self-esteem.

Action-Oriented: Break down your short- and long-term goals into weekly targets. This gives you the satisfaction of meeting your short-term goals and offers you a regular opportunity to assess whether your goals are still the appropriate course of action for your larger picture. It's much easier to make adjustments to your game plan than to quit. Quitting means you will have to live every minute of every day knowing that you failed to live up to your potential, and trust me, the pain of regret is far worse than the pain of discipline.

Realistic: Don't buy into the fantasy of fad diets and diet products. Instead, educate yourself about diet and exercise. This can also be as simple as finding someone around you who has been able to lose weight and keep it off. These people are valuable resources because they can help provide motivation and support, and they understand how to set realistic goals.

If you don't have immediate access to someone who can help you, here is an example of a realistic goal you can set:

If you are used to drinking 12 cans of sodas every day, it is unrealistic to assume you will give up drinking pop altogether by tomorrow. This is one reason why so many diets fail. Diets typically ask you to make drastic and immediate changes to your lifestyle instead of making subtle changes that are more sustainable long-term.

In this instance, it's much better to slowly reduce your intake. You can say something like, "I'm only going to drink 8 pops every day instead of 12." This helps because you're not giving up all of the things you enjoy. It will be easier for you to stick with your game plan this way, and small goals like this add up to big results over time. The average 12 ounce can of soda contains 143 calories and 40 grams of sugar. Thus, just by cutting back on your consumption, you will not only end up saving a lot of money, but you will also end up losing over ONE POUND OF FAT EVERY WEEK and 59 pounds of fat a year!

Timed: Set a deadline for when you want to see your goals accomplished. This will help motivate you to action. A goal without a deadline is a "wish or a want," not a goal. Goals must be timed and have an objective timetable.

Use the Be SMART system of goal setting as a template to help create your own weight-loss plan, and remember that you deserve success.

Congratulations on everything that you have gone through to get to this point, and as we are coming to the conclusion of our time together, please remember to stay in touch.

I wish you all the best in your endeavors!

Your Friend and Trainer,
Scott Schmaltz

Please Stay in Touch

I would love to hear your story!

Over the course of more than ten years, I have personally worked with hundreds of clients. Each and every client has created a very memorable and moving experience for me. No one has been forgettable or unimportant, and I would love to continue to be a part of your own personal, weight-loss story and to share in your successes.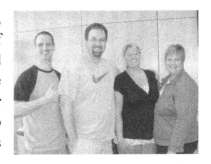

I am planning to write another health and fitness weight-loss book, and I firmly believe that your own story and experiences have meaning and importance beyond measure and can be used to help touch the lives of thousands of others just like you.

I would love to hear from you about the kinds of successes and struggles that you have had both your own weight-loss journey and throughout your **Six-Week Body Challenge**.

Please feel free to email me with your story! Also make sure to send plenty of high-resolution photos so I can see your progress too. (Please send all photos and emails to: scott@customworkoutvideos.com.)

Once I get a chance to look over your stories and experiences, I would be happy to contact you and discuss your experiences, see if we can help others using your amazing story, and personally answer any questions that you may have about health and fitness. I will do my best to personally reach out to each and every one of you. I can't wait to hear back from you!

By the way:

My attorney did, however, mention that I should tell you that all photos and any other materials ("Materials") submitted to me become my ("Scott D. Schmaltz") sole and exclusive property and cannot be returned at any time.

By submitting Materials, you are agreeing that I may, but am not obligated to; use the Materials in connection with any of my future works, in any way, in any medium, worldwide, in perpetuity. Further, you warrant that all Materials are 100% original and do not violate the right of privacy or publicity of, or constitute a defamation against, any person or entity; that the Materials will not infringe upon or violate the copyright or common law rights or any other rights of any person or entity; that there are and will be no encumbrances, liens, conditions or restrictions whatsoever upon or affecting such Materials; and that you are at least 18 years of age and the person depicted in the Materials. You also agree to indemnify me, my publishers, and any other broadcasters and entities that I work with for any and all damages and expenses (including reasonable attorney's fees) arising out of any breach or failure of the warranties made herein.

About the Author

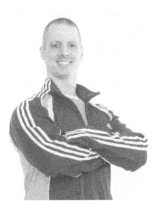

Scott Schmaltz is also the co-author of *The Couch Potato Diet* © **Family Edition** with author Gregory J.E. Ladas (www.TheCouch PotatoDiet.com).

Scott Schmaltz is a veteran of the fitness industry, with more than 10 years of experience. He holds a board certification as a Holistic Health Practitioner from the American Association of Drugless Practitioners (AADP), a degree in nutrition from the Global College of Natural Medicine (GCNM), and seven certifications in personal training and rehabilitation (NASM, NCSF, APEX, and 4 from NIHS in Senior Fitness and post surgery rehab). Scott is the creator of Precision Fitness and Custom Workout Videos, which produces and sells online exercise and nutrition videos (CustomWorkoutVideos.com).

Scott has run personal training departments and corporate wellness programs for companies including Gold's Gym, Snap Fitness and Health Partners Insurance Company. He is passionate about helping people improve their lives by improving their self-image and their spiritual self, and by reshaping the limiting beliefs that prevent weight loss.

For more information, join up with Scott on Facebook, where he shares lots of great exercise tips, recipes, insights and updates at: http://www.facebook.com/scottschmaltz.fanpage

About the Editor

Addie Zierman is a freelance copywriter based in the Twin Cities, MN with a background strongly rooted in both business and creative writing. She began her career as a catalog copywriter and then spent several years writing online help and user's guides for a prominent software company. She also recently received her Master's in Creative Writing from Hamline University, where she honed her writing craft.

As a freelance writer and editor, Addie has done everything from musician bios to web pages. She knows that while the skills required to excel at both technical and creative communication differ in some ways, the real "magic" happens when you combine the clear precision of business writing with the fresh, innovative nature of creative writing. It is this authenticity that she brings to all of her writing and editing projects.

To learn more about Addie's writing and editing services, visit her website: www.addiezierman.com.

BUY A SHARE OF THE FUTURE IN YOUR COMMUNITY

These certificates make great holiday, graduation and birthday gifts that can be personalized with the recipient's name. The cost of one S.H.A.R.E. or one square foot is $54.17. The personalized certificate is suitable for framing and will state the number of shares purchased and the amount of each share, as well as the recipient's name. The home that you participate in "building" will last for many years and will continue to grow in value.

Here is a sample SHARE certificate:

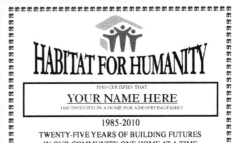

HABITAT FOR HUMANITY

THIS CERTIFIES THAT

YOUR NAME HERE

HAS INVESTED IN A HOME FOR A DESERVING FAMILY

1985-2010

TWENTY-FIVE YEARS OF BUILDING FUTURES
IN OUR COMMUNITY ONE HOME AT A TIME

1200 SQUARE FOOT HOUSE @ $65,000 = $54.17 PER SQUARE FOOT
This certificate represents a tax deductible donation. It has no cash value.

YES, I WOULD LIKE TO HELP!

I support the work that Habitat for Humanity does and I want to be part of the excitement! As a donor, I will receive periodic updates on your construction activities but, more importantly, I know my gift will help a family in our community realize the dream of homeownership. **I would like to SHARE in your efforts against substandard housing in my community!** *(Please print below)*

PLEASE SEND ME _____ SHARES at $54.17 EACH = $ $_____

In Honor Of: _____

Occasion: (Circle One)   HOLIDAY   BIRTHDAY   ANNIVERSARY

        OTHER: _____

Address of Recipient: _____

Gift From: _____ *Donor Address:* _____

Donor Email: _____

I AM ENCLOSING A CHECK FOR $ $_____ PAYABLE TO HABITAT FOR HUMANITY OR PLEASE CHARGE MY VISA OR MASTERCARD *(CIRCLE ONE)*

Card Number _____ Expiration Date: _____

Name as it appears on Credit Card _____ Charge Amount $ _____

Signature _____

Billing Address _____

Telephone # Day _____ Eve _____

PLEASE NOTE: Your contribution is tax-deductible to the fullest extent allowed by law.
Habitat for Humanity • P.O. Box 1443 • Newport News, VA 23601 • 757-596-5553
www.HelpHabitatforHumanity.org